Sex Surveyed, 1949–1994

Feminist Perspectives on the Past and Present
Advisory Editorial Board

Sex Surveyed, 1949–1994

From Mass-Observation's 'Little Kinsey' to the National Survey and the Hite Reports

L IZ S TANLEY

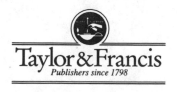

Taylor & Francis
Publishers since 1798

| UK | Taylor & Francis Ltd., 4 John St., London WC1N 2ET |
| USA | Taylor & Francis Inc., 1900 Frost Road, Suite 101, BRistol, PA 19007 |

First published 1995.

A Catalogue Record for this book is available from the British Library

ISBN   0 7484 0367 1 (cloth)
ISBN   0 7484 0368 X (paper)

Library of Congress Cataloging-in-Publication Data are available on request

Photoset by Stephen Cary

Printed by SRP Ltd, Exeter

Contents

Contents

Acknowledgements

Without Dorothy Sheridan's unparalleled knowledge of the Mass-Observation Archive, and Joy Eldridge's great ability to guide and support researchers, this book, and indeed the work of many other researchers, would not have been completed. Jane Haggis typed the 'Little Kinsey' manuscript and deciphered more of the handwritten parts than I was ever likely to; the best typist and transcriber that I have ever known, I am sure that she prefers her own research at the University of Adelaide. Janet Finch gave me the solitude of her house so that I could read and think about the original 'Little Kinsey' manuscript – our task-master the Higher Education Funding Council owes her! My thanks for routines and cuddles to Mrs W. Rochester, Diva Jessye Norman, Professor Alfred Schutz, Mr Precious Mackenzie, and, last but by no means least, St Thomas Aquinas. This book, like so much else, is for Sue Wise, for the last 22 years and the next, with all my love.

Mass-Observation, 'Little Kinsey' and the Sex Survey Tradition

Introduction

'Little Kinsey' – Some Feminist Issues and Interests

'When I was 20 I didn't know a thing, and I went to see our parson . . . He . . . said 'Do you grow marrows, George? . . . Well, you've got to pollenize marrows . . .', and he showed me how it was done'

' . . . some can go through a full life and never think nothing about sex, but they're very very few. I have done'

'I think it is very unpleasant . . . If I'd known what it was like before I got married I would never have married'

'I agree with it [pre-marital sex]. It's to try people out — you never want to buy a pig in a poke'

' . . . you can see women that's never been happy, and men that's never had a woman. And they look as if they're going seedy, they have that green and mouldy look'

'better for them [children] to live with one parent than in an unhappy home with two'

'Sex isn't very nice . . . Yes, it can be harmful, it can ruin a woman's inside as easy as pie, ruin any girl's innards, intercourse can'

'I am very satisfied. I have been very clever or very lucky in my choice of partner'

'If only he had made love to me instead of using me like a chamber pot'

'I shouldn't think they're [homosexuals] human . . . I mean animals don't do that, I shouldn't think'

These quotations are taken from 'Little Kinsey', a sex survey carried out in 1949 by an organization known as Mass-Observation. For a number of reasons, 'Little Kinsey' must count as one of the most important pieces of British

3

sex research, and it has particular interest and significance when looked at with a scrutinizing feminist eye.

'Little Kinsey' was the first national random sample survey of sex to be carried out. It was influenced by the 1948 Kinsey study of American male sexual behaviour, which used more 'unconventional' interviewing methods than 'Little Kinsey'. However, although 'Little Kinsey' was carried out within a British random sample survey tradition, it made innovative use of ideas about random sampling and computerized methods of quantitative data analysis, not least because at the same time it also challenged this emergent orthodoxy by insisting on the equal validity and importance of coupling the quantitative results with qualitative data. 'Little Kinsey' thus not only predates the apparently pioneering national random survey approach of the British 'National Survey of Sexual Attitudes and Lifestyles' (published in 1994) by some 45 years, it predates the 'alternative' methodological concern with qualitative research and analysis, and it also anticipates by some 40 years the attempts of 'triangulation' to utilize different kinds of data within a common epistemological frame. Consequently, its successes, and perhaps even more its failures, have interesting methodological and epistemological reverberations for social science. There are also aspects of this that have particular resonance for feminism

'Little Kinsey' was carried out in the context of Mass-Observation's concern, between 1937 and 1949, with investigating all aspects of social life in Britain. Mass-Observation had been set up as a popular radical alternative form of social science. Overarching the different research approaches, methods and techniques that it used, Mass-Observation articulated a highly distinctive epistemological and methodological approach that has, perhaps surprisingly, a good deal in common with that of 1990s feminist social science. Such commonalties are striking particularly when met in the context of Mass-Observation's 'outsider' oppositional relationship to mainstream social science of its day, a relationship that parallels in fascinating respects that of feminism from the 1970s to the 1990s. 'Little Kinsey' both adheres to and departs from the more general Mass-Observation approach in consequential ways, particularly with regard to its treatment of women's lives and experiences, and its use of different kinds of data and different kinds of research 'voice' or stance.

Mass-Observation investigated many aspects of British everyday life – smoking behaviours, local customs, dance crazes, behaviour on holiday, reading, shopping, cinema-going, anti-Semitism and much more – and it rapidly became a familiar topic of discussion, in newspapers and magazines, on the radio, and even during the very earliest television broadcasts. Mass-Observation also looked in detail at life in the north-west of England, in 'Worktown'. This was Bolton, in the late 1930s a cotton town still in the midst of depression, but none the less a town that revolved around work, paid and unpaid, permanent and casual, and where there was a long tradition of women as well as men being employed full-time throughout the life-course.

Indeed, for Mass-Observation, women were central to what one of its Worktown projects called the 'Economics of Everyday Life'.[1] And in parallel with its Worktown research, Mass-Observation also looked at Worktowners on holiday in 'Seatown', in pre-war Blackpool as the prime location of the annual week away for working-class northerners with its attractive mixture of holiday license and highly regulated propriety;[2] and it was here that the first Mass-Observation research concerned with the complex and interesting relationship between 'the sexual' and 'the social' took place.

At the start of the 1939–1945 war, Mass-Observation carried out research for the government through the Home Intelligence Department of the Ministry of Information, including on air-raid precautions (ARP), the evacuation of children, the blitz, rumour, and the effectiveness of various government campaigns. Even after it ceased being associated in this way with the government, Mass-Observation's wartime research remained both very varied and highly characteristic of its particular methodological stance, and it included research on sexual behaviour, particularly concerning the spread and prevention of venereal diseases and changes in the national birth-rate.

By the end of the war, many people who worked in or headed voluntary and statutory organizations concerned with marriage, childbirth, and birth control within and outside marriage, were increasingly aware that the war had brought with it major changes to sexual attitudes and behaviour, with attendant effects on the national birth-rate. Rather than guessing what these changes might consist of from the highly selective evidence then available, some of them wanted more exact and less impressionistic information. Some people were also aware of the research that Alfred Kinsey was carrying out in America[3] and wondered whether something similar might be carried out in post-war Britain. It was in this context that one of them, Marjorie Hulme of the Society of Friends Council on Sex, first tentatively proposed that Mass-Observation should carry out such research. Eventually the project came to fruition with a group of these people acting as Advisors to Mass-Observation, including David Mace from the Marriage Guidance Council, Gilbert Russell of the Church of England Moral Welfare Council, Eva Hubback, a feminist and writer on demographic issues,[4] Cyril Bibby, a human biologist and writer on health education issues,[5] psychologist Clifford Allen, who wrote on 'sexual perversions and anomalies,[6] as well as Marjorie Hulme herself.[7] The resulting research was widely known, in the press and academic writings as well as within Mass-Observation, as 'Little Kinsey'.

By 1949, when 'Little Kinsey' was carried out, Mass-Observation was in transition from its earlier political and methodological radicalism to its later incarnation as a commercial market-research organization. 'Little Kinsey' was centrally involved in this transition. From what was initially intended to be an observational and largely ethnographic study of public forms of sexual and quasi-sexual behaviours – including 'getting off', prostitution, courtship and canoodling – 'Little Kinsey' changed rapidly over a few weeks into a national representative sample survey of sexual attitudes. The result offers an unparalleled insight into British sexual mores as these had been influenced by changes associated with, perhaps even caused by, the war, including the new expectations that women had about their lives, that young people had of what they thought was acceptable sexual behaviour, that people in general had of the relationship between marriage and sexual pleasure and between marriage and childbirth.

Both 'Little Kinsey' and Mass-Observation's earlier research on the birth-rate[8] pinpoint many women's dissatisfactions with marriage, indeed with heterosexuality, in their then-current forms. Marriage for many women brought with it sex of a kind all too often unwanted, not enjoyed and merely endured, but at the same time marriage also meant public acceptability, a division of labour ensuring women's economic survival, and, above all else, children. Mass-Observation's research on the birth-rate had shown that women were busy re-fashioning the very structure of 'marriage and the family'. Its 'Little Kinsey' research shows equally clearly that there were reasons for this beyond the wish to control family size and thus the family economy: love, passion, desire, pleasure, disgust, distaste, hate, despair; powerful feelings indeed lie behind the statistical headcounts of all sex surveys. Because of 'Little Kinsey's' textual reliance on extended quotation, however, they are also there, visible on its pages, illustrated by the quotations that stand at the head of this Introduction.

In spite of being a British 'first' in the field of sex surveys and receiving a good deal of newspaper and radio publicity at the time it was carried out, 'Little Kinsey' is now largely unknown even among specialist researchers. It has become a 'lost' foremother to the British sex survey tradition, remembered only in brief acknowledgements that there had been such a study and with little now realized about its approach, its scope, the large sample involved, and its pioneering attempt to combine quantitative and qualitative data. Its 'disappearance' occurred for complex reasons: the planned book was completed but not published until now; this seems to have been related to the key researchers involved deciding that their analysis of the data and resultant overall argument was unsatisfactory; and relatedly, Mass-Observation was at the time undergoing great organizational and methodological changes. Nonetheless, and as this book shows, 45 years on 'Little Kinsey' is still a fascinating and methodologically challenging piece of work, and, substantively, it and the Mass-Observation tradition of sex research within which it was located tell us an enormous amount about the sources and processes of social and economic change occurring at that time. Even a cursory glance at national statistics over the period 1945–1995 demonstrates the enormous changes that have occurred in British women's lives and consequently within men's lives also, with married women's mass (re)entry into the labour market, the planning and control of fertility, changes in the duration and dissolution of marriage, and concern about women's sexual pleasure, among them. The stock in trade of gender-aware researchers only now after much argument and insistence from feminism, each of these factors was in its first hints and beginnings delineated, discussed and theorized in Mass-Observation's sex research; no small accomplishment.

Herein lies yet another reason for a lively feminist interest in this research. Mass-Observation was interested in behaviours and issues that currently engage feminism. It explored many aspects of women's lives and experiences and noted the interpersonal as well as structural inequalities involved in a way highly similar to feminism; it was centrally concerned with what we would now call gender as the lynch-pin of social structure; and its interest was operationalized in a broad research approach that has many points of similarity with the methodological position advanced by feminism. Yet in spite of these things, Mass-Observation was not a 'feminist' organization and in some respects its organizational framework and structure of decision-making and control were antithetical to women's interests and organizational equality. The conundrum here is how to explain these enormous similarities and also how to pinpoint and analyse the points of difference; as I shall suggest later, neither is as straightforward as might be supposed.

There are other reasons why feminism should take note of 'Little Kinsey', concerning the fact that what had been intended as an observational study quickly turned into a survey, and, relatedly, the greatly changing status of survey-based research at the time that 'Little Kinsey' was carried out. Pre-war there had been a 'survey movement' in Britain, albeit one neither so powerful nor so far-reaching as in America; and this had promoted the use of the survey approach to the investigation of demographic areas and the amelioration of the social problems located within them. Alongside this, entangled in its activities and yet not completely synonymous with it, was the development of ideas about sampling, random sampling specifically, and with later important theoretical developments that made random sampling a practical possibility for survey researchers. The need for information on a large-scale during the 1939–1945 war encouraged the use of such ideas and practices and also promoted the development of mechanical, and then computerized, aids to the analysis of the resulting data. The immediate post-war period saw the growth of both sampling theory and also mechanical and computerized methods of analysis, initially particularly in the burgeoning of the activities of commercial market-research organizations. 'Little Kinsey' was both 'in', and yet not quite 'of' this emergent and soon-to-be canonical emphasis on 'the survey'. As I discuss in Section Three, pre-war the term 'the survey' had held a number of different meanings and research practices, while, after it, increasingly it meant not only quantification, but quantification in the particular form of random sampling; and the stance underpinning 'Little Kinsey' shifted uneasily but fascinatingly between these two meanings.

Neither in the 1940s and early 1950s, nor indeed at any point subsequently, has one and only one methodological approach had total dominance within any of the social sciences. By the 1950s, random surveys located in a highly positivist framework were gaining a canonical status within sociology in particular – but of course 'a canon' can and typically does coexist with a variety of alternatives within a discipline, precisely the situation at that time with both positivism in general and random sampling and the survey as a particular method of investigation. Relatedly, a part of the growing canonical status of the survey as a method lay in popular views of science and the association with it of mathematics in general, counting in particular, as a means of deriving 'the facts' about social life and using these to produce social policy. Such a view of social science is of course implicit in Cartesian ideas about science generally; however, it was made explicit by the need of government during the war for large amounts of superficial information delivered quickly, economically and accurately – the forte of the survey. It was in such a context of the need for information that Mass-Observation's birth-rate study (published in 1945) was carried out just before the 1947 Royal Commission on the Population was set up to investigate the same set of issues – and of course a similar need for information to inform the policies and practices of a number of voluntary groups occasioned 'Little Kinsey' itself. Through the 1950s and 1960s, it was to a very large extent the fetishizing of the survey in and by the mass media, coupled with publicity about the work of commercial market-research organizations, that underpinned popular beliefs about – and in – survey research; the situation in the social science disciplines was much more varied and contested, and consequently much less dominated by the survey as the method of investigation. None the less, these popularized media versions of survey research have been important in forming popular views about 'British society', 'what other people are like', 'what is happening', 'normal behaviour' and so forth, and also in informing, to put it no stronger, public policy formation and the discourses that surround this.

It is in my view important, crucial even, for feminism to develop a critical, but nuanced and appreciative, understanding of the historical origins and development of 'the survey' and its complex relationship with science and with government. 'The survey' now is too socially important to ignore, too politically respectable not to take seriously, and intellectually engages too many aware and concerned people, many feminists among them, be dismissive of. During the initial period of the development of its canonical importance in Britain, Mass-Observation in general and 'Little Kinsey' in particular played interesting parts. Perhaps in a sense they were on the side-lines to the key developments in theory and the major organizational and academic shifts that accompanied this, but in another sense Mass-Observation was centrally involved, because along with many other research organizations it was concerned with the processes of putting these ideas into practice, sometimes in greatly modified form because of the exigencies of actual research. Moreover, 'Little Kinsey' itself represents the eye of the storm of change: at one point in time a planned observational study, but only a few weeks later a completed national random survey.

The results of surveys appear, and are certainly frequently presented within the mass media, as providing incontrovertible and scientifically proven facts about social life and human conduct. This assumption and legitimacy of 'science' has become attached particularly to the national random sample survey with its claims of representativeness and generalizability. Some 'voices' within the feminist critique of social science methodology (in the sense of a general research framework and approach) and method (in the sense of specific research techniques or tools) have at times almost uncritically assigned qualitative approaches to the 'good' end of a spectrum and quantitative approaches and methods to the 'bad' as masculinist in assumptions, practices and knowledge-claims. However, a more consistent and intellectually more important strand in the feminist critique has been directed towards 'science' itself, its assumptions, approaches, knowledge-claims, its popular and academic status, as well as the gender composition of its organization structures and publishing frameworks and controls. This critique has been concerned with the practices and claims of 'scientism' regardless of method in the narrow sense, and has included its qualitative as much as its quantitative forms. The argument and approach I have adopted here is consonant with this latter wider set of feminist concerns with the organizational apparatus and outputs of science, and eschews any moral dichotomization of method. Thus, my concern with the context within which 'Little Kinsey' is located, and indeed to an extent with 'Little Kinsey' itself, is a concern with this important historical 'moment' in the development of the survey and its transition from its earlier meaning of an analytic overview to its new meaning of quantification within the framework of random sampling. More than this even, it is also a concern with the shift from 'a survey' as a broad humanist concern with the investigation of social problems in order to effect their amelioration, to a specific scientific concern with investigation as such.

While these shifts and transitions in 'the survey' have a general trajectory and pattern, they also have a trajectory and pattern in relation to the *sex survey* as a particular variant. The national random sample-based sex survey in Britain has offered apparently objective scientific facts about the sexual behaviours and sexual attitudes of the general population; and such surveys have also offered to whole generations bench-marks against which particular individuals could, and did, measure themselves, to find themselves conforming to or being deviant from the general pattern of 'rates of intercourse', 'rates of orgasm', 'use of birth control', 'levels of marital satisfaction', and so forth. More than this, within the results of these researches, there has been an implicit bench-mark against which one entire group of people were constrained both to measure themselves *and* to find themselves different and so wanting. The bench-mark, as I shall discuss later in Section One in relation to a number of British sex surveys, was formed by male sexual experience, behaviour and attitudes; women's difference from this was scrutinized, delineated, theorized and explained, but always as women's departure from an assumed male norm in sexual terms. This has considerably over-problematized women's behaviours, attitudes and 'differences', and equally considerably it has under-problematized those of men. In addition, and perhaps more importantly in an analytic sense, it has *assumed* male behaviour and experience, and assumed them in a particular and highly stereotypic form, rather than *investigated* the extent to which men, as well as women, might depart from public gender stereotypes. Perhaps paradoxically, as I shall argue in Section Three, it has been largely as a consequence of the development of feminist ideas that male sexuality, sexual behaviour and sexual attitudes have been 'normalized' by being displaced as an assumed norm.

In these introductory remarks I have made reference to some of the great sources of interest that not only 'Little Kinsey' but also Mass-Observation itself has for contemporary feminism. In the rest of Section One I discuss this in more detail, looking at the emergence and organizational structure of Mass-Observation, its epistemological and methodological stance, its sex research over the period 1937–1949, the wider context of sex survey research from the 1940s to the 1990s, and the largely implicit theorization of 'sex' and its relationship to the social embedded within these sex surveys. The text of 'Little Kinsey' then follows in Section Two. Section Three discusses the Mass-Observation theorization of sex in 'Little Kinsey' and outlines similarities and differences between it and the feminist investigation and theorization of sex in the surveys carried out by American researcher Shere Hite. I argue that 'surveying sex the feminist way' has a good deal in common with surveying it the Mass-Observation way.

Notes

1   This project is discussed in Liz Stanley (1990a) 'The archaeology of a 1930s Mass-Observation project'; and (1992) 'The economics of everyday life: a Mass-Observation project in Bolton'.
2   See here the excellent collection by Gary Cross (Ed.) (1990) *Worktowners at Blackpool: Mass-Observation and popular leisure in the 1930s.*
3   Kinsey's *Sexual Behaviour in the Human Male* was published in 1948.
4   See Mace (1944, 1946, 1971). Eva Hubback was Principal of Morley College from the late 1920s to the 1950s as well as being a key figure in the feminist organization the National Union for Equal Citizenship and one of the founders of the Family Planning Association. She published a number of books on demographic issues, including *Population Facts and Policies* (1945), and *The Population of Britain* (1946).
5   Cyril Bibby wrote on human biology and health education topics, including on 'morality'; see Bibby (1944) *Sex Education: A Guide for Parents, Teachers and Youth Leaders.*
6   Clifford Allen published on a variety of related topics from a predominantly Freudian viewpoint. For example Allen (1952) *Modern Discoveries in Medical Psychology* sees sex and hate as the two central human drives, and perceives an almost absolute gendered division of characteristics and sexual behaviours which positions sex as a priori heterosexual unless something 'goes wrong', and then this can be 'cured'. See also Allen (1940), (1950), (1958) and (1962).
7   See Mass-Observation Archive Topic Collection (MOA-TC) 12 Box 2, File A: Progress report of 28 January 1949 from Len England to Hugh Cudlipp at the *Sunday Pictorial* for a discussion concerning the advisors.
8   Mass-Observation (1945) *Britain and Her Birth-Rate;* this research is discussed later.

Chapter 1

Britain, by Mass-Observation

Mass-Observation was founded in 1937 by Tom Harrisson, Charles Madge and Humphrey Jennings as a mass popular sociology that would carry out sufficiently detailed empirical research to form an 'anthropology at home' – the aim was to know the details of ordinary people's lives 'at home' at least as well as anthropologists knew the lives of those 'abroad'. At this time, sociology's mainstream was concerned with large-scale, usually historical, comparative theorizing; while its minor stream of small-scale empirical studies remained largely peripheral and failed to take seriously the specificities of place, time and locality that were for Mass-Observation absolutely crucial to understanding British society. Harrisson, returning to Britain in 1936 from ornithological and anthropological trips abroad, and with a wide-ranging, albeit iconoclastic, interest in the social sciences, insisted that sociology did not even treat Britain as a 'savage civilization' (the title of Harrisson's first book, a maverick study of 'cannibals' in Melanesia[1]). He argued that sociology treated Britain as an unknown land in which it had little interest, an approach that was mirrored in the stance of Britain's government towards its people. Thus, for its founders, the 'mass' in Mass-Observation had a quite different contemporary meaning than is now familiar: neither undifferentiated nor lacking in individuality, but rather indicative of the need for democracy and equality.

Mass-Observation was founded around the events of the 1936 Abdication Crisis, which demonstrated to the then-*Daily Mirror* journalist Charles Madge the extent of the government's ignorance of and contempt for the opinions of the people by whom it was elected. He appealed for like minds to join him in investigating 'public opinion' as this cohered around crises in an open letter published in the *New Statesman*. Both Harrisson and Humphrey Jennings[2] responded to this letter, with crises becoming an important topic in *Britain*, one of Mass-Observation's earliest publications.[3] All three shared a commitment to a broadly left-wing stance, particularly the ethos of Left Book Club circles.[4] Madge and Jennings in particular were also interested in surrealism, Jennings in relation to film-making and Madge in relation to poetry, although Harrisson's *Savage Civilisation* shows that he too was influenced by surrealist ideas about form. Surrealism appealed because of its juxtaposition of incongruities, but also its subordination of linear 'rational' and temporal structures to the multi-centred and fragmented flow of events when conceptualized from the viewpoints of the myriad of people who compose them (a set of ideas that long predate postmodernist theory of course). All three men realized that such ideas could be used with political intent to disturb the orthodoxies of 'knowledge' enshrined in the assumptions and practices of the social science establishment, including by means of the pivotal role assigned to mass-observers in the organization's National Panel: large numbers of 'ordinary' people who were recruited and trained to become proficient observers of their own and other people's lives.

Mass-Observation's founders thus shared ideas about unknown Britain and the need to establish an anthropology at home, they held similar views about the need to investigate public opinion and to relay the views of the governed to the government, and they wanted to explore the political ramifications of surrealism's power to disturb. They also shared a distinctive understanding of the relationship between an observer and what they observed, summed up in the Mass-Observation description of its mass-observers as 'subjective cameras'. The social science establishment insisted that scientific – i.e. 'objective' – observation was observer-independent, so promoting the view that any trained and objective scientist would observe precisely the same thing as any other. In contrast, the emergent Mass-Observation nailed a radically different set of colours to its research mast, arguing that all observation was tied to, and marked by, those who carried out this observation. Its first publication, *Mass-Observation*,[5] proclaimed the 'subjective cameras' view, while its account of the Coronation Day of George VI, *May 12: Mass-Observation Day-Surveys 1937*,[6] does so to greater effect by actually showing within its pages the very different knowledges produced by different observers of Coronation Day in different places and from different classes. Certainly *May 12* occasioned extremely hostile responses from mainstream social scientists,[7] who seemingly understood little of the epistemological challenge Mass-Observation was mounting, seeing its activities as merely a failed version of their own 'objective' and 'scientific' one.

The distinctive Mass-Observation understanding of the relationship between observers and observation was in large part influenced by the socialism of the organization's founders, their conviction that 'the masses' were important and their views should be consulted and taken seriously. For Harrisson and Madge in particular, the social location of an observer conditioned not only what was observed but also how it was observed. For them, a truly useful 'science of ourselves' would be something produced, not by an academic élite, but rather by the mass of people: thus, mass-observation.[8] However, this is not to propose that there were no methodological or other differences of understanding and approach between the key figures of Harrisson and Madge. These differences extended beyond their very diff-erent personal styles – Harrisson's arrogance and bombast as well as his magnetism and drive, Madge's introspection as well as his affability and charm. Perhaps the most important difference concerns the overall aims and purposes of Mass-Observation. For Harrisson, Mass-Observation's activities were the route to founding a new synthetic social science that would transcend the growing divisions and boundaries between the different social sciences, while for Madge the aim was more simply the collection and presentation of facts about the mass of people.[9] Both agreed that fact should proceed theory – in today's terminology, they promoted 'inductive theorizing' and rejected a 'deductive' approach in which theory proceeded research – but alongside this went Harrisson's conviction that eventually this approach would produce social theory of the order and power of Darwin's on evolution.

The organizational structure of Mass-Observation was an apparently simple one. Charles Madge set up and ran, from Blackheath in London, a 'National Panel' of volunteer mass-observers, initially predominantly male but, as time went on, including increasing numbers of women, recruited via press and radio reports of Mass-Observation's activities. Members of its Panel wrote responses to monthly 'directives', which were sets of characteristically-phrased questions on diverse topics. Tom Harrisson lived and worked in Bolton – Worktown – and encouraged other people, again predominately men, to do the same for shorter or longer periods of time, recording as writers or artists or researchers their observations of the ordinary everyday life of a northern mill town. However, in practice matters were considerably more complex than this, even during the first phase of Mass-Observation's life, from its founding in 1937 through to the outbreak of war.

First, in London, as well as recruiting and organizing the National Panel, Charles Madge also raised money, often from private companies, to carry out specific pieces of research, for example on shopping behaviours and reading habits, and these funds were used to subsidize more politically motivated or otherwise 'meaningful' research, for example on anti-Semitism. Both kinds were carried out by a combination of paid observers[10] and a floating population of volunteers. Second, the National Panel was often used within the commercially-funded pieces of research. Third, regardless of whether activities were carried out by Harrisson and others in Worktown, through the National Panel, or by paid and volunteer observers around the London office, reports of them were relayed back to a variety of overlapping audiences through duplicated 'Bulletins' of two or three sides to Panel members, in printed 'file reports' for internal circulation but also for selected external contacts. Then, after war started, they were circulated in a newsletter called *Us*[11] that had a more varied mailing list. And fourth, in November 1938, Harrisson and Madge changed organizational places and Madge went to Worktown to carry out a very different and more straightforwardly 'academic' style of investigation than had characterized Harrisson's approach, with a smaller and more professionalized group of researchers looking at the 'Economics of Everyday Life'.[12]

In terms of popular response, Mass-Observation's activities were widely reported in the local and national press, on radio and even on the new television broadcasts, and occasioned much interest. Both Harrisson and Madge, in rather different ways, were skilled at obtaining the maximum publicity possible, Harrisson through personal magnetism as well as force of personality and the deliberate contentiousness of many of his statements;[13] Madge because of his journalistic contacts and interpersonal skills. By and large the popular response was highly favourable: Mass-Observation was news, and interesting. The social science response is by no means so simple to describe.

The initial academic reaction was largely supportive of Mass-Observation's attempt to closely investigate British society. Bronislaw Malinowski, then a key figure in social anthropology, became Mass-Observation's treasurer, although his essay about Mass-Observation in *First Year's Work*[14] mixed compliment with criticism of what he saw as its lack of objectivity. Other British academics, such as the social psychologist T.H. Pear and the economist John Jewkes (both at the University of Manchester) among others, were less publicly involved but supported Mass-Observation by providing limited funds and also visits from students during vacations. However, as the large differences between Mass-Observation's approach to research and that of most social science academics became clearer, a considerably more critical stance was adopted, as with the reviews of *May 12* by T.H. Marshall, Marie Jahoda and Raymond Firth,[15] of *People In Production* by Margaret Bunn,[16] and more complexly of Mass-Observation's entire project in the edited collection *The Study of Society*,[17] which originated largely as a countering response to Mass-Observation's iconoclastic methods and its equally iconoclastic methodological stance and pronouncements.

In the initial stages of the 1939–1945 war, Mass-Observation continued its by then characteristic range of activities, although many of these now had a 'war flavour' to them, looking at, for example, air-raid precautions (ARP) and 'careless talk' about the war, while later research looked at the 'home front', rationing, and, towards the end of the war, carried out a number of pieces of work concerned with venereal diseases which I shall discuss in more detail later. Behind the scenes Tom Harrisson negotiated, through Mary Adams, then head of the Home Intelligence Service, for Mass-Observation to carry out research of direct use to the government, and in 1940 Mass-Observation was associated with 'Team B' of the Wartime Social Survey.[18] This relationship lasted until organizational changes occurred within the Survey, ending in 1942. During this period Mass-Observation reorganized the range of its research activities in response to the war by, for example, encouraging Panel members to write diaries for the duration of the War and reinstating the collection of 'day-diaries' as part of the thematic directives sent to Panel members.[19]

Over the period of the war many of those who had been closely associated with Mass-Observation's pre-war activities were called up or volunteered to enter the armed services or engaged in other warwork, including

Tom Harrisson and Len England in 1942, while Charles Madge's connections with the organization had by then already become much looser.[20] However, others saw their involvement with Mass-Observation as warwork in its own right, and Mass-Observation unsuccessfully asked the government for exemption from call-up for its staff.[21] Mass-Observation remained highly research active, with the area of its greatest activity constituted by varied investigations of public morale and changes to this produced by the events of the war, including the evacuation of children, the blitz, and the Dunkirk evacuation.[22]

As the war ended, former Mass-Observation personnel returned to Britain; Tom Harrisson remained in the Far East until autumn 1946, while Len England returned to become office manager, and the roles of John Ferraby (one of the organization's 'backroom' writers), Bob Willcock (office manager during most of Harrisson's absence) and others who had remained in England took a different turn, given the changing composition of the people involved in the organization. New people with very different ideas about social research joined Mass-Observation. Some of these newcomers, with an interest in computer-based methods of analysing large amounts of data from interviews, became important in the 1949 'Little Kinsey' research. The result was a meeting of different traditions of research and its analysis that, around 'Little Kinsey', eventuated in the demise of Mass-Observation in its original form and the rise of a new professionalized market-research organization, 'Mass-Observation Ltd'.[23]

As my earlier remarks about the gender composition of the National Panel and the early Worktown research suggests, there are interesting issues to be explored about the role of women within this first phase of Mass-Observation, for in the current Mass-Observation National Panel project run from the Mass-Observation Archive at the University of Sussex there are now considerably more women than men.[24] However, beyond the initial dearth of women in the Panel, and the infrequency with which women, compared with men, made the transition from Panel membership to working on the ongoing research projects such as Worktown,[25], Mass-Observation makes a considerably better show in its research treatment of women's lives and experiences,[26] as some examples demonstrate. A pre-war example concerns the 'Economics of Everyday Life' project headed by Charles Madge in Bolton from November 1938 to late 1941, which saw women as central to household finances through their independent paid labour and their control of family spending and saving, and thus also as central to the local economy. A war-time example is Mass-Observation's research on women's warwork,[27] in particular in the three areas of the recruitment of women into the labour force, 'dilution' of the traditional labour force, and demobilization at the end of the war, for, by focusing on everyday life and what women thought and said, Mass-Observation asserted women's lack of power, their difficulties in combining domestic and paid work, the monotony of warwork, and the expression of male hostility to their presence in local workplaces. An example, which I discuss in more detail later and which is drawn from its research at the end of the war, is Mass-Observation's investigation of Britain's falling birth-rate, in which it pinpointed with accuracy trends – such as women's wish for smaller numbers of children, and for a life and work outside of the home – which became apparent to mainstream social science only years afterwards. In each of these examples, Mass-Observation not only centred women's lives and experiences, but also recognized and explored problems as women saw them, thereby giving its research a quite remarkable ability to understand and predict when compared with other contemporary research on similar topics.

Just as interesting as the gap between the frequently high level of gender-awareness in Mass-Observation's research and the low level of such awareness regarding its own organization is the part played by gender factors in the movement from the 'old' to the 'new' styles of Mass-Observation research. In a book published in the early post-war period, Dennis Chapman, who had worked on the 'Economics of Everyday Life' research, argued that quantitative methods avoided the research mystique of the qualitative ('it's an attitude of mind') because they were composed by a specific set of techniques and skills that could be taught and learned, and which were thus more consonant with a reforming radical stance within the social sciences.[28] One of the means by which women were marginalized or subordinated in, for example, the first phase of the Worktown research, was through their exclusion from 'knowledge', of how to do what the Mass-Observation researchers were there to do. Exclusion, marginalization and subordination were somewhat different outcomes to the same set of processes, which hinged on the pre-eminent organizational position of Harrisson and Madge, deference to their ideas and programmes of activities, and the great deal of centralized control that they exerted;[29] these factors were coupled in Worktown with Harrisson's highly particular mixture of sexual flirtatiousness, control and Puritanism.[30] Such interactional dynamics and organizational structures changed, first with Harrisson's absence and the development of a very different central organizational style, then with the war-time and post-war entry into Mass-Observation of women who, through their warwork, had become highly skilled in the analysis of large-scale quantitative forms of social data: they not only had 'knowledge' but technologically *better* knowledge. This was a phenomenon by no means confined to Mass-Observation, for much of the social research conducted during the war had been carried out by highly skilled and trained women who became highly competent in newly developed techniques, including the theoretical ones connected with sampling and the practical ones concerned with the use of computers.[31]

Notes

1   Tom Harrisson (1937) *Savage Civilisation*.
2   Jennings's particular interests lay with film-making as a form of representation,

and his activities soon began to separate from those of Harrisson and Madge. During the war Jennings made films for the Government's Documentary Film Unit; he was killed in a climbing accident in 1950.

3   Tom Harrisson and Charles Madge (1939) *Britain, by Mass-Observation*.
4   Victor Gollancz, publisher and distributor of 'the Left Book Club' as well as of the publishing company of Gollancz itself, provided Mass-Observation with generous advances for much of its earliest research – a number of its planned books were to have been published by Gollancz, and generous advances on these funded the research.
5   Charles Madge and Tom Harrisson (1937) *Mass-Observation*.
6   Humphrey Jennings and Charles Madge (1937) *May 12: Mass-Observation Day-Surveys*.
7   Thomas Marshall (1937) 'Is Mass-Observation moonshine?'; Marie Jahoda (1938) 'Review of Mass-Observation and of May 12'; Raymond Firth (1939) 'An anthropologist's view of Mass-Observation'.
8   See here Madge and Harrisson (1937) *Mass-Observation*, also Charles Madge and Tom Harrisson (1938) *First Year's Work*.
9   Madge and Harrisson (1937) *Mass-Observation* p.1.
10 These paid observers clustered around the embryonic national office but carried out investigations in different parts of the country as well as in London.
11 Mass-Observation's file reports, including related documents, are available on microfiche through most major libraries.
12 See Stanley (1990a) 'The archaeology of a 1930s Mass-Observation project' and (1992) 'The economics of everyday life: a Mass-Observation project in Bolton'.
13 Harrisson had a large number of influential friends and acquaintances who pulled strings, opened doors and also often provided finance for his ventures.
14 See Bronislaw Malinowski (1938) 'A nation-wide intelligence service', in Madge and Harrisson (Eds) *First Year's Work*, pp.81–121.
15 See note 7 above.
16 Margaret Bunn (1943) 'Mass-Observation: a comment on *People in Production*'.
17 Frederick Bartlett, Morris Ginsberg, Ethel Lindgren and Ralph Thouless (Eds) (1939) *The Study of Society*.
18 'Team A' was concerned with survey research, while members of 'Team B' carried out a variety of qualitative kinds of investigation.
19 See MOA File Reports 510, 523A, 598, 619, 621, 689, 773, 774, 847, 868, and 2181 on the wartime diaries.
20 See Stanley (1990a) 'The archaeology of a 1930s Mass-Observation project'; Charles Madge engaged primarily in research on savings and spending while involved in this Worktown project, and later did similar research during the war for John Maynard Keynes (see Madge, 1943).
21 See MOA-FR 1450.
22 See the File Reports on morale (over 250), on propaganda (over 150) on air raids (over 100) and air-raid precautions (ARP) (over 60), as well as those on the blackout (10), the evacuation of children (over 40), rumour (25), fears about the invasion of Britain (24), and Dunkirk (6).
23 Mass-Observation Ltd still exists, although in 1992 it became a division of the British Market Research Bureau Ltd.
24 See Dorothy Sheridan (1992) 'Ordinary hard-working folk: volunteer writers in Mass-Observation, 1937–50 and 1981–91', (1993) 'Writing to the Archive: Mass-

Observation as autobiography', and also David Bloome, Dorothy Sheridan and Brian Street (1994) 'Reading Mass-Observation writing', for interesting discussions of the current Panel project and its relationship to Mass-Observation of the 1930s.

25 Celia Fremlin did so, and was later responsible for Mass-Observation's (1943) *War Factory*; while the writer Naomi Mitchison was a Panel member, wrote detailed reports of night-time London during the blitz for Mass-Observation and also wrote for the organization a wartime diary later published as *Among You Taking Notes* (Mitchison, 1985). These were redoubtable, self-assured upper- and middle-class women: all characteristics likely to be necessary to cope with the class-reinforced masculinist urbanity of Madge and sexist bombast of Harrisson.

26 For an overview, see the papers in 'En/Gendering the Archive: Mass-Observation Among the Women' *Feminist Praxis* 37/38.

27 See Penny Summerfield (1992) 'Mass-Observation on women at work in the Second World War'.

28 Dennis Chapman (1955) *The Home and Social Status*.

29 However, the position of Gertrud Wagner is interesting here, for she had been on the periphery of the ethnography- and interview-based Marienthal study of male unemployment (Jahoda-Lazersfeld and Zeisel (1933) *Marienthal*) and then later involved in a variety of similar research when she came to Britain. This included as an interviewer on the influential Pilgrim Trust (1938) project *Men Without Work*. She joined the Worktown 'Economics of Everyday Life' project; and it is also likely that she helped to complete writing the text of Mass-Observation's best-known book, *The Pub and the People* (Mass-Observation, 1943).

30 An example of this is Harrisson's attempt to enforce 'separate spheres' as a sign of respectability in the otherwise extremely unrespectable Davenport Street house that was Mass-Observation's Bolton headquarters, together with his sexual interest in, verging on sexual harassment of, some of the women researchers there.

31 For interesting discussions of the historical origins of the survey and developments in its form, see here Bulmer's introduction to, as well as contributions in, Bulmer (1982b), particularly Marsh (1982b); see also Marsh (1982a).

Chapter 2

From Observing to Surveying, from Seatown to 'Little Kinsey'

In March 1949, Mass-Observation produced an internal memo that was headed 'Directive for penetrative work on sex survey'.[1] The term 'penetrative' was used because many of the ideas about research held by Oscar Oeser, a social psychologist based at the University of Stirling, had entered Mass-Observation terminology via published reports of his methodologically highly-innovative study of long-term unemployed (female as importantly as male) ex-jute workers in Dundee.[2] 'Functional penetration' described the research practice in which a group of 'outsiders', a mixed team of social psychologists, sociologists, anthropologists and others, took on 'inside' employment and social roles so as to conduct their research by 'penetrating' the group or community being studied. Oeser was clear that 'outsiders' could understand only insofar as they became insiders and so came to know what insiders know, with social scientists then subsequently using their outsider's theoretical ideas to analyse the insider factual knowledge they had thus gained.

Oeser's ideas were different from the notion of ethnography being developed at this time in two important ways. One was Oeser's recognition that no community could be properly understood when looked at from one standpoint only – and thus his emphasis on research conducted by a team, with members including both men and women, who would take up different activities and occupations, and doing so in different social contexts. The other was Oeser's related conviction that no community could be understood properly without cross-disciplinary, indeed inter-disciplinary, work and understanding. Certainly in the late 1930s, when Oeser's research was carried out, the boundaries between the social science disciplines were far less marked than they are today, including methodological barriers. Nonetheless, growing differences of approach were discernible; and Oeser among a group of other influential social scientists – including Philip Sargant Florence and Wilhelm Baldamus at Birmingham, and Adolf Lowe at the LSE and Manchester University – in contrast promoted a vision of a synthetic social science centred on economic sociology;[3] and Oeser's work articulated a method for empirical research consonant with this theoretical and organizational position. These ideas struck powerful chords with the protagonists of Mass-Observation. Not only was Harrisson – in spite of his loudly announced disdain for both institutional social science and respectability – always on the look out for 'respectable' academic support for Mass-Observation, but also Oeser's notion of 'functional penetration' put into practice in a coherent social science framework aspects of Mass-Observation's own independently constructed approach.[4]

Within this approach, Mass-Observation proposed that an observer had to become in some sense an insider to what was observed: not necessarily a direct member of a specific group or conversation, but certainly a 'knowing' member of the wider social collectivity within which these activities took place. It associated the research of individual observers with that of a large number of others, each observing from their own particular standpoints. That is, it saw research into any community or activity as an essentially collaborative activity, not necessarily in the details of being carried out but certainly in bringing together and using many different accounts in writing about such research.[5] It also recognized that the informal aspects of research – just living and being in the context of study – could be as important in gaining knowledge as those activities defined as 'research' in the narrow sense. Relatedly, it made a fundamental distinction between obtrusive and unobtrusive research techniques and opted very firmly for the latter, eschewing direct questioning and instead focusing on 'follows' and 'overheards', in which interesting persons or groups were trailed, and overheard conversations were recorded in as much detail as possible. In doing so, it focused on ordinary life, on the rhythms and patterns of the ordinary 'at home', which it argued remained largely unknown to social science research. And Mass-Observation also insisted that detailed observation and description were the heart of research, and that only when all pertinent observation had been completed could there be any systematic theory-building.

These characteristic elements of Mass-Observation's approach can in today's terminology be seen as an embryonic epistemological position,[6] one which encapsulated political and ethical principles put into practice within the organizational structure and methodological procedures of Mass-Observation. There is something of a contradiction here, however, for Mass-Observation combined a levelling radicalism in its stance on observation, of the mass-observer being and living in the research context conducting naturalistic forms of research within the everyday, together with a considerably more conventional elitism in which a specialist group (Mass-Observation's central personnel) produced analytical knowledge from the descriptions provided by 'their' mass-observers. *May 12* is actually a good instance of this, with its apparent fragmentation of experience but its actually highly active central researcher/writer presence, selecting in particular descriptive instances of Coronation Day to produce a pattern chosen by the writers[7] and not by the observers; and in this *May 12* had considerably more in common with mainstream social science than its reviewers recognized. This particular contradiction, as I have termed it, between one aspect of its principles and practice and others, was later to become crucial with regard to 'Little Kinsey', for, as I shall argue in more detail later, it was this attempt to centre the research experience of the mass-observers within a text actually written from the researcher/writer's standpoint that produced the problems discerned by the writer of 'Little Kinsey' (Len England) and which led to its failure to be published.

This characteristic Mass-Observation approach is interesting in other ways also, for feminist epistemologies too are strung between similarly con- tradictory aspects, regarding the representation and analysis of *women's* lives and experiences, but within a text actually produced from the standpoint of the *feminist* researcher. This is particularly noticeable regarding what has been called the 'standpoint' epistemology,[8] which is variously termed the 'feminist standpoint' and the 'women's standpoint' position, as though women and feminists were somehow synonymous groups. However, it is a contradiction that can also be discerned in other feminist epistemological positions, not because of theoretical or other inadequacies, but rather because 'settling' such issues requires the prior 'settling' of all the major epis- temological issues of the social science: no easy matter now – and of course no easy matter for Mass-Observation during the 1930s and 1940s either.

The 'Directive for penetrative work on sex survey' follows the wider pat- tern of Mass-Observation's (by 1949) highly characteristic approach, and sets out a programme for three kinds of research to be carried out. The first and most important was for observational research and was to include at least three dance-halls visited a number of times during a seven-day period, the 'worst' public houses, and some pornographic bookshops. The second was concerned with providing back-up statistics and was to include the collection of arrest figures for 18 offences, including abortion and infanticide, sex under age, indecent exposure, prostitution and living off prostitution, and a variety of sexual 'offences' between males, to be collected from the local police sta- tion; VD figures from the local Health Department or clinic; and figures for affiliation, maintenance and separation orders from the Magistrates Court. The third, closely related to the observational research, was for two types of interviews to be conducted: formal interviews with 'executives', including clergy from the main denominations, a probation officer, local councillor, police officer, doctor and bar-keeper; and a large number of 'informal' ones where the person involved would not know that they were actually being interviewed rather than just having a casual conversation. The formal inter- views were to focus on views about changes in sexual morality and 'bad spots', and the informal ones on courtship, picking up, love-making[9] and sex- ual relationships, including affairs.

Traces of this initial research approach can still be seen within the text of 'Little Kinsey' even though its main focus changed markedly soon after this directive was produced. Initially the plan had been for the whole study to consist of such 'penetrational' work in the two contrasting communities of

'Churchtown' (Worcester) and 'Steeltown' (Middlesborough). However, what finally resulted was very different, for this initial characteristic Mass-Observation style of approach became subordinated to three surveys that were carried out only a few weeks later but which are not even mentioned in the directive: (1) a national random representative survey of 2000 people – the 'Street Sample'; (2) a randomly selected postal survey of 1000 cach of clergy, doctors and teachers – the 'Opinion Leaders' survey; and (3) a postal survey of Mass-Observation's 1000 strong National Panel of mass-observers.

Thus in 1949, in the wake of Kinsey's *Sexual Behaviour in the Human Male*, and following its own earlier research on VD and on the falling birth-rate, Mass-Observation carried out the 'Little Kinsey' research.[10] The research was paid for by the *Sunday Pictorial* and was in part published in a series of articles that appeared in this newspaper during July 1949.[11] As well as these short articles, written by *Pictorial* journalists from material supplied by Mass-Observation, it was also intended to publish a Mass-Observation book. Negotiations with the intended publisher, Allen and Unwin, took place, at the advice of one of Mass-Observation's external advisors, David Mace, with Stanley Unwin himself. A draft text was completed and its receipt acknowledged by Allen and Unwin on 1 June 1949.[12] However, the book was not published until now, although the typescript that forms Section Two of this book still exists in the Mass-Observation Archive at the University of Sussex.[13] A plan for the projected book[14] was sent to the external advisors in July 1949. Most of the chapters proposed in this plan exist in final typescript, although a few exist in manuscript, while some chapters are mentioned else-where in Mass-Observation documents using chapter numbers and titles that are different from this plan. These complexities exist because both earlier and later versions of the proposed book seem to have existed; however, I have foll-owed the July 1949 plan, as the typescript more closely corresponds to this than to any other reference in the Archive.[15]

Why 'Little Kinsey' was never published is a puzzle, to an extent still unsolved. The writer of the typescript, Len England, in 1949 Mass-Observation's office manager and a considerable presence in the organiza-tion, cannot now remember why it never appeared;[16] and Allen and Unwin's records contain no information concerned with the projected book. However, there are clues which, when pieced together, suggest that the book's non-appearance was connected to wide-reaching organizational changes occur-ring within Mass-Observation. In 1949, Mass-Observation was a still well-known research organization, although its public profile was nowhere as high as it had been from 1937 through to about 1942–1943. As I noted earlier, Mass-Observation had been set up as a radical force in British social and political life; it is therefore all the more ironic that 'Little Kinsey', in method-ological terms the most 'respectable' of Mass-Observation's major pieces of research, heralded the end of the old-style Mass-Observation that had so per-sistently – and successfully – thumbed its nose at scientific respectability. Around a series of internal changes, the organization's old-guard, and more importantly its founders, surrendered their financial and managerial interest in Mass-Observation, and the new guard took what then became 'Mass-Observation Ltd' into a new life as a commercial market-research organization.

Central to these internal changes was the wartime development and use of the computer and the post-war availability to research organizations of computer facilities. There are some brief mentions in Mass-Observation documents associated with the 'Little Kinsey' project about the organization's computer, a Powers machine,[17] and these take on significance when placed in the context of Mass-Observation's changes of personnel and its newer members' more 'scientifically respectable' approach to social research as an exercise in the quantification of attitudes. The result was that what had been originally envisioned as a piece of the basically qualitative research style pioneered by Mass-Observation became a large-scale national representative sample survey.[18] The technology was available and there had been a major shift in the intellectual climate generally as well as within Mass-Observation, a shift that is discernible in the considerably wider post-war move into surveys and quantification within the social sciences, in sociology especially.

References to the earliest version of the sex research project[19] show the intention to emphasize public forms of sexual behaviour: in dance-hall and public house 'pick-ups', prostitution, and holiday-making public license. This derived from central tenets of Mass-Observation's research position and paralleled its earlier 1930s research in Blackpool.[20] The Blackpool research utilized many of what became standard features of a Mass-Observation investigation, particularly direct observation supplemented by 'overheards' and 'follows', but not direct questioning apart from ordinary conversations, which only the observer knew were part of a research exercise (its 'informal interviews'). The Blackpool research focused on dance-halls, cafés, the prom and the pier and their many attractions, parks, the beach, and also under the pier; and it emphasized not only the differences between the relative decorum of these places in daytime and the license that characterized them at night, but also pointed out that actually rather little of this license involved penetrational forms of heterosexual sexual behaviour. This was somewhat to the discomfort of Blackpool's civic notability when such reports appeared in the press, for it was the sexual promise of Blackpool that attracted many of its vast numbers of working-class holiday-makers. A long passage at the end of Chapter 10 of 'Little Kinsey', which describes observations of public sexual behaviour in Blackpool, illustrates this point. The original passage in the Worktown collection suggests that little of this behaviour involved intercourse;[21] however and interestingly, this particular statement has been omitted from the quotation in 'Little Kinsey', making the behaviour seem different from what it actually was.

'Little Kinsey' was concerned with sexual attitudes and not with sexual behaviours. This point was repeatedly made in negotiations with the *Sunday Pictorial* and with the project's advisors. In an early letter to Marjorie Hulme discussing the possibilities of researching sex, Len England emphasized that it would not be possible to use '*the direct methods used by Professor Kinsey . . . in this country*',[22] and the same point is also stressed at various points in the text of 'Little Kinsey'. As well as pointing up the comparative 'respectability' of Mass-Observation's approach in dealing with the general public and avoiding any complaints and controversy about the national 'Street Sample' part of its research, this emphasis on attitudes and not behaviours should be seen as part of the 'new guard' adherence to the ethos of commercial survey research.

British commercial market-research organizations of the time were greatly influenced by the social psychology-derived approach of similar American organizations, aided by the presence of the British Institute of Public Opinion (BIPO), the British branch of Gallop, founded in the late 1930s. The emphasis was on tapping the 'attitudes' of those questioned, on the premise that people's minds are composed by sets of pre-existent attitudes, to butter or margarine, Conservative or Labour, sex or chastity, that transcend the specifics of particular meals, particular elections, particular sexual encounters. Relatedly, such an approach assumes that actual behaviours are a product of these pre-existing attitudes: the person who expresses prejudiced attitudes, for example, will be a person who behaves in prejudiced ways, or, more simply, the person who says they will vote Labour or Conservative will indeed do so. Mass-Observation from its inception challenged what it considered to be the over-simplistic understanding of attitudes held by market-research agencies,[23] a stance shared with social scientists of a more radical methodological persuasion.[24]

As well as measuring attitudes, market-research organizations of the post-war period worked within an emergent orthodoxy concerning random representative sampling procedures as the basis of survey research. Certainly up until the immediate post-war period, the term 'survey' could imply any one of a number of rather different methodological approaches. It could entail a broad overview using equally broad-brush documentary evidence, as for example in Terence Young's survey of the development of Becontree and Dagenham.[25] It could involve basically qualitative studies, as for example in Len England's letter to Brian Murtough about a Mass-Observation sex survey that would use a combination of observational and 'penetrational' methods[26] – that is, what in today's social science language would be called ethnographic or participant observation research. And it could involve a detailed quantitative approach, but one which did not use a random sampling procedure, as for example with many of the city and regional surveys carried out as part of the 'survey movement',[27] such as the Pilgrim Trust study of the effects of long-term employment in six towns, *Men Without Work*.[28]

However, ideas about random representative sampling gained wider currency in Britain during and immediately after the war, not least through the work of the Wartime Social Survey. A number of Mass-Observation staff joined the Wartime Social Survey, with one of them, Geoffrey Thomas, later becoming the Director of its post-war transformation into the Government Social Survey. Also in the immediate post-war period there was considerable contact between academic social scientists, Mass-Observation and commercial survey agencies, including through meetings organized by Political and Economic Planning (PEP), headed at this time by Charles Madge until his appointment to a professorial chair in Sociology at the University of Birmingham in 1950. Post-war, Tom Harrisson largely retained his pre-war championing of observational methods and attention to everyday conversation, and also his insistence that a worthwhile discipline of sociology must be concerned with the minutiae of everyday life.[29] However, his absence from Britain until 1946 meant not only that Mass-Observation survived a long time without his daily involvement, but also that other staff members developed independent research and writing skills and methodological and epistemological ideas to go with them;[30] and also a sense of themselves as no longer in thrall to what had seemed, pre-war, to be the immeasurably superior knowledge, drive and sophistication of Harrisson. These changes to the nexus of relationships that composed the national office of Mass-Observation, along with the employment of new members of staff influenced by the new ideas about surveys and sampling, and the increasing dominance of these ideas in the commercial and academic research scene, all contributed to the final 'Little Kinsey' emphasis on attitudes and its move away from an observational and 'penetrational' approach.

The key areas of sexual attitudes that 'Little Kinsey' investigated include: how people found out about the 'facts of life'; whether they had had anything that could be called 'sex education'; if they did, who had provided it, and who should provide it for the children of the 1950s; what people thought of the use of birth control; what their views were of marriage and the place of children within it; whether they thought that divorce should be easily available as a means of ending unsatisfactory marriages; their views of 'extra-marital relations' (a term confusingly used about both sexual relationships before marriage and also adulterous relationships); and how they saw prostitution. Chapters on each of these topics appear in the text of 'Little Kinsey', and in each of them there is an interesting and, in survey terms, highly unusual attention to variance within responses: to *differences* by sex, by age, by class, by region and so forth. That is, rather than focusing on generalities, analytical attention is directed towards difference and complexity. 'Little Kinsey's' key data certainly comes from the investigation of the attitudes of people in each of the three samples used. However, enough of the earlier spirit and approach of Mass-Observation was retained for 'the numbers' to be supplemented by observational material from the comparative studies of public sexual behaviours in 'Churchtown' and 'Steeltown', and the private sexual behaviours of 'Homosexual Groups' (actually one group of gay men). And in addition, respondents frequently failed to observe the attitude/behaviour distinction, instead responding in terms of their own and other people's behaviours. Thus, although Tom Harrisson's 'Preface' to 'Little

Kinsey' (reprinted in Section Two with the rest of the text of 'Little Kinsey') stresses that it is an investigation of attitudes only, 'Little Kinsey' in fact includes a good deal of fascinating material about sexual behaviour as well.

Notes

1 See MOA:TC12: Box 2, File 15 Box 3/15.
2 Oscar Oeser (1937) 'Methods and assumptions of fieldwork'; and (1939) 'The value of team work and functional penetration as methods in social investigation'.
3 See in particular the discussion in Adolf Lowe (1935) *Economics and Society*.
4 The interest was a mutual one; Oeser visited Worktown at least once, and was in fairly close contact with Harrisson in the pre-war phase of Mass-Observation's life.
5 And the study of Coronation Day 1937 in *May 12* represents the apotheosis of this.
6 By epistemology I mean a theory of knowledge itself, of what this is, how it is produced and by whom, who knowers are, how competing knowledge-claims are adjudicated and by whom. That it was recognized as such is indicated by the work done in drafting a 'Mass-Observation' methodological textbook, an uncompleted project that had importantly involved Mass-Observation's 'back-room writer', John Ferraby, who wrote up many Mass-Observation projects.
7 *May 12* was written by Humphrey Jennings and Charles Madge from the accounts of many mass-observers, with Madge providing the final edit of the book (personal interview, Charles Madge with Liz Stanley, 23 March 1988).
8 See Sandra Harding (Ed.) (1987) *Feminism and Methodology* for definitional work in naming the standpoint position; and also Stanley and Wise (1990) 'Method, methodology and epistemology in feminist research processes' for a discussion that is critical of the taxonomical approach to feminist epistemologies. A useful overview of current debates is provided by Kathleen Lennon and Margaret Whitford (Eds) (1994) *Knowing the Difference: Feminist Perspectives in Epistemology*.
9 'Love-making' probably meant just that, a set of courtship behaviours that did not necessarily include genital sexual behaviour.
10 See Len England (1949) 'Little Kinsey: an outline of sex attitudes in Britain'; and (1950) 'A British sex survey'.
11 The fliers for the series appeared on 19 June and 26 June, and the articles themselves appeared on 3 July, 17 July, 24 July, 31 July 1949.
12 See MOA:TC 12 Box 2/K.
13 In the order of the edited manuscript, these are MOA:TC 12 Box 3/A, 3/B, 3/C, 3/D, 3/E, 3/F, 3/G, Box 4/A, 4/B, 4/C, 4/D, 4/F, 4/G, and 4/E.
14 See MOA:TC 12 Box 3/15D; and also MOA:TC 12 Box 2/C, letter 24 August 1949 from Len England to Marjorie Hulme.
15 See MOA:TC 12 Box 3/A, undated draft outlines.
16 Personal interview, Len England with Liz Stanley, 22 August 1990.
17 For example, MOA:TC 12 Box 2/G, letter 24 January 1949 from Len England to Eva Hubback.
18 See for example MOA:TC 12 Box 2/A, letter 10 December 1948 from Len

England to Brian Murtough, the features editor of the *Sunday Pictorial.*
19   See MOA:TC 12 Box 3/15.
20   Like most of the other planned books on Worktown to have been published by
      Gollancz, the Blackpool study never appeared although there are a considerable
      number of drafts of planned chapters and sections, various of which appear in
      Cross (Ed.) (1990) *Worktowners at Blackpool.*
21   Apart from the National Survey, in the sex surveys discussed later the terms 'sex'
      and 'intercourse' are used interchangeably but usually without being defined.
      The assumption seems to be that all 'sex' is intercourse, i.e. the penetration of a
      vagina by a penis. However, this is a researchers' assumption only, for none of
      these surveys investigate in any detail precisely what behaviours compose 'sex'
      and 'intercourse' and whether, and for whom, there may be more going on than
      penetrational forms of behaviour alone. There is, however, a kind of half-recog-
      nition that matters are more complex than this, as indicated by the appearance
      in all of them of the term 'petting' to stand for all other sexual practices, but
      which are then separated off from 'sex' itself.
22   See MOA:TC 12 Box 2/B, letter 4 March 1948 from Len England to Marjorie
      Hulme.
23   For example, in Harrisson and Madge (1939) *Britain, by Mass-Observation.*
24   See, for example, the chapter in Bartlett *et al.* (Eds) (1939) *Study of Society* by
      T.H. Pear 'Some problems and topics of contemporary social psychology'; Oscar
      Oeser, 'The value of team work and functional penetration as methods in social
      investigation'; and P.E. Vernon 'Questionnaires, attitude tests, and rating scales'.
25   Terence Young (1934) *Becontree and Dagenham.*
26   See MOA:TC 12 2/A 10 December 1948.
27   Alan Wells (1936) 'Social surveys and sociology'.
28   Pilgrim Trust (1938) *Men Without Work.*
29   Tom Harrisson (1947) 'The future of sociology'.
30   For example, the various interesting methodological writings produced by John
      Ferraby, noted above.

Chapter 3

Mass-Observation's Sex Research, 1937–1949

Although it is conventionally seen as purely 'private', people actually come to understand sexual conduct (that is, sexual feelings and thoughts, sexual behaviour, and also talk about all of this) in a social and shared, rather than an 'internal' and individualized, context. Precisely what 'it' consists of, who can legitimately engage in 'it' and with what kind of partners, what are normal and deviant varieties of 'it', how 'it' meshes with other behaviours and other relationships, what all of this means and the feelings involved: all of these things are learned about as part of a more general process of growing up and finding out, using mis/information culled from a wide variety of sources. Moreover, the construction and understanding, and indeed the doing, of 'it' also varies between different cultures (for example, in some societies penetrational forms of heterosexual sex are considered the last refuge of the inadequate lover, while in others this defines all that 'it' can legitimately be) and in the same culture over time (for example, in Britain now 'it' is conventionally done in private, by adults of 'opposite' sexes, without onlookers, and in bed usually at night; while in the early Victorian era social investigators could tut-tut at 'it' being done in public, by children, in varying combinations of the sexes, with onlookers, in the streets, and at a range of times).

However, alongside present-day British convention about the apparently private nature of sex, much sexual behaviour actually takes place in, and very much more is represented in, a highly public context. We are accustomed to seeing kissing and canoodling, 'getting off', 'flaunting' modes of dress, seductive glances and gestures and movements; and also of course media representations of all these, and much more, on billboards, in newspapers and on television, in magazines and on radio, in novels and poetry, and in music. Pinpointing precisely how the 'non-sexual' and the 'sexual' are defined and how the boundaries between them are perceived and indeed lived are all highly complex matters. This is in part because 'love' and 'sex', and sometimes of course hate and sex, relate, overlap and separate in highly complex ways. It is also in part because we live in a representational world in which cars can conjure up sexual encounters, champagne bottles can represent male ejaculation, and actual sexual behaviour can be experienced as hard work for little reward. And it is also because 'sexual' thoughts and feelings can infuse situations, persons and objects that are apparently and, on the surface, completely 'non-sexual', and anyway what is experienced as 'sexual' can differ considerably between people.

In the discussion that follows I indicate this complexity, problematizing the term most often used by placing it, 'sex', in inverted commas. I do so particularly because not only in popular usage but also in the majority of the post-war surveys the behaviour involved is on the one hand assumed to be entirely synonymous with 'intercourse', as heterosexual and penetrational; but, on another and more implicit level, greater complexities are hinted at by researchers' use of the term 'petting' to indicate a wide range of other erotic sexual practices. Thus, the hints of the complexities and problematics of 'sex' can be discerned in the major sex surveys, but in their brief glimpses of *people's* actual behaviours, and which are largely if not entirely hidden by *researchers'* assumptions that sex, intercourse and heterosexuality are entirely synonymous.

Mass-Observation's investigations of sex focused on the realm of public sexual conduct. Such a focus derived from the way in which its investigators worked, and this in turn came from the methodological stance that Mass-Observation pioneered, which I outlined earlier. That is, from its inception and in all the major trajectories of its research, the emphasis was on investigators and Panel members learning how to observe for themselves in great – and unaccustomed – detail, and also to record this in equally great detail; and this observation was in the form of direct observation and/or 'overheards', and the recording of indirectly gained information was explicitly warned against. Public life and conduct was Mass-Observation's almost defining concern.

This emphasis on direct observation/knowledge came from Mass-Observation's (and particularly Tom Harrisson's) understanding of the nature of knowledge-production: all observers are 'subjective cameras' and therefore it is crucial for sociologists and other social investigators not to rely on second-hand reports, but rather explicitly to link the necessary subjectivity of an observation or series of observations to the interpretation and theor-ization of the particular observer. Relatedly, from the same stance came the determined focus on behaviour rather than attitude: behaviour, and particularly 'habit' (repeated behaviour), was what people actually did, and thus what Mass-Observation considered social investigation should be concerned with, while attitude was the product of convention and social pressure and in its view often bore a very indirect relationship indeed to actual behaviour.

The practical research stance that resulted from these emphases was both highly distinctive and also extremely threatening to the 'scientific' status of both the academic social science establishment and to the market-research organizations then in the process of becoming established. The increasingly negative reaction of social science to Mass-Observation has already been referred to, and it focused on what were perceived as Mass-

Observation's methodological 'failures'. The post-war criticisms from market-research organizations, and particularly Mark Abrams's swingeing attack on Mass-Observation's failure to use conventional survey methods and sampling procedures,[1] seized upon Mass-Observation's methodological difference from an assumed random sample survey norm. However, by the time Abrams's critique appeared, the Mass-Observation approach that had been the object of his ire effectively no longer existed, although Mass-Observation Ltd had become a direct competitor with BIPO, for which Abrams worked – and it is in relation to this commercially competitive context as well as the pre-war history of his relationship with Harrisson and with Mass-Observation that Abrams' critique must be evaluated.

The distinctiveness of Mass-Observation's investigations of sex can be seen in the three main kinds of research on this topic that the organization undertook before 'Little Kinsey': on Worktowners in Blackpool, on venereal disease, and on the falling birth-rate. I discuss these Mass-Observation projects before looking at the post-war sex survey research to which 'Little Kinsey' must be related and, in a sense, against which it must be compared.

Worktowners in Blackpool

The Blackpool investigations were a by-product of the Worktown study. Initially Tom Harrisson lived in Worktown and worked in a variety of temporary or casual jobs there. He was joined, following the formation of Mass-Observation, by a changing group of people, some local to Worktown, more from London, from the universities, and a sizeable proportion of whom were later associated with the London-based part of the organization and the commissioned research projects it carried out as its 'bread and butter' way of earning money. Worktown was Bolton, a town where both men and women worked full-time in the labour market throughout the life-course, predominantly in its textile mills – always supposing there was such employment to be had. For one week of the year, traditionally known as 'Wakes Week', Bolton and many other northern towns emptied out. The prime desired destination for Boltonians was Blackpool, a northern Mecca with its beach, tower, prom, cafés and bars, side-shows and arcades, its boarding houses and hotels, and its promise of excitement and a good time away from home and work. By and large Worktowners were drawn by the attractions of *the resort* and not by the seaside itself.

Mass-Observation's investigators followed Worktowners to Blackpool, often literally, and to everything they did while there, including the particular 'good times' of which the younger and unattached holiday-makers were in search. The Blackpool investigations included promenading, the funfair, side-shows and 'freaks', eating in cafés and going to shows, boarding-house life, and it particularly noted the enormous disruption of everyday patterns of behaviour and time and movement. In Mass-Observation writings,

Worktowners in Blackpool are characterized around the disruption of the usual rhythms of life, their continual movement between rest and restlessness, no sooner settling into one activity than moving in search of another in a different place.

It is around this movement between stasis and activity that sex is discussed, in particular through the contrast between the individual holiday-maker and 'the mob', the restless crowd in public places, being observed eating, drinking, promenading, dancing, in pubs and after closing time. Another contrast here is that between the 'sexual legend' and the reality of Blackpool: a putatively sexual environment where reality is anticlimax, figuratively and literally, for most of the sex that takes place is married, legitimate and in private, and the large amount of public sexual behaviour is typically associated with 'not going the whole way'. The public aspects of Blackpool sexual conduct included dancing and chatting, 'going out', flirting and pickups, groping on the beach, knee-tremblers and the prostrate bodies of couples on the beach at night. The research concludes that both private and public sex was little different from in Worktown apart from in the varied contexts and times of occurrence, except that 'at home' was known and familiar and so, for many people, provided more opportunities for the illicit.

Venereal Disease

In December 1942, Mass-Observation questioned its Panel members regarding their attitudes to venereal disease and its treatment,[2] sending out a directive asking them to record their 'general beliefs and feelings about VD' to which 125 replies were received. The report notes that most Panel members disassociated themselves from 'traditional' attitudes to VD: they were opposed to secrecy and to moral and religious approaches that saw VD as some kind of retribution. Panel members generally deplored the lack of knowledge, secrecy and social stigma surrounding the subject, pointing out that this prevented many people from seeking the medical treatment they needed as well as stopping them from learning about and using preventatives. Of the minority of Panel members who supported traditional attitudes, the women who did so were less dogmatic and more open to contrary viewpoints than the men. The majority of Mass-Observation's Panel members, and women even more than men, adopted a liberal stance that saw education as the most efficacious long-term remedy, while more men than women favoured compulsory notification by doctors of VD and state-regulated prostitution and brothels. However, nearly a fifth of female and just under a tenth of male Panel members reported knowing nothing at all about VD; and the bulk of the report is an account, using verbatim quotations, of the nature of ignorance of the subject and the mythology that sees it as akin to the common cold: easily caught in public places, from shared towels and toilet seats and even by touching the same handrail as someone suffering from it.

In January 1943, Mass-Observation's 'Report on public attitudes to VD'[3] detailed the results of surveying a sample of 435 predominantly working-class Londoners about their general attitudes to VD and also to the widely reported debates regarding the government's proposed Regulation 33B, which was intended to make notification and treatment compulsory. In carrying out the survey, male interviewers interviewed men and female interviewers women. Under five headings (general attitudes, Regulation 33B, opinions about VD publicity, suggested treatment, and conclusions), the report notes that the large majority thought the problem should be brought into the open, approved of the publicity given to it, and thought people should be given more information. Within the sample, twice as many men as women expressed embarrassment at talking about the subject and at reading the press articles, with their unaccustomed public use of terms such as intercourse, contraception and VD itself. Women sample members were more approving of the articles than men, and oddly this is ascribed to their greater degree of ignorance, although there is nothing in the report that supports this contention beyond the fact that fewer of the women had read the press articles than men, while the men who did not approve of them did not want their wives or children being able to read about 'things like that' and more men than women objected to any increase or extension to the publicity. It is actually more consonant with the findings from both of Mass-Observation's VD investigations to see the women sample members as simply more liberal on such topics than the men: more men than women were in favour of the proposed Regulation 33B; and those who objected included more women than men, and they did so for two reasons – an objection to compulsion, and a conviction that compulsion would drive the problem 'underground' again.

Most of the sample members, both women and men, saw VD as an ordinary disease that should be treated as such, socially as well as medically (rather than as the product of divine retribution). However, at the same time a good many people – and more women than men – thought that if information was given to children this would make the problem worse by encouraging early sexual experimentation. A significant proportion of the sample did not know about any preventatives that could be used and which would work, in the main because of 'you catch it much like a cold' ideas about how VD was contracted. However, a very large majority[4] wanted more instruction on the subject of its prevention and treatment, with predominantly women favouring education (through lectures, classes, radio and special films), with again predominantly men favouring compulsory notification and treatment and the setting up of government approved brothels.

In March 1943, Mass-Observation produced an 'Extract of news-quota questionnaires',[5] which dealt with a very much smaller sample's reactions to the question 'Have you seen any of those VD advertisements in the papers?', the research for which was carried out in February 1943. This work was probably done to confirm the general findings of the January 1943 survey and the

'Report on public attitudes to VD', that people approved of the publicity and that fewer women than men had seen it. However, although this second earlier finding was confirmed, a considerably lower proportion of both men and women in this smaller sample approved of the publicity.

Overall, then, Mass-Observation's VD research took a quantified form, making use of percentages, tables of results and so forth. However, it also retained a focus on the National Panel, first carrying out Panel research and then using the results from this to set the parameters of subsequent work. Thus while perhaps not entirely characteristic of Mass-Observation's research style, its VD research is nonetheless fairly typical of that important sub-stream of its work, often but not always commercially funded, which was carried out using street samples; it departs from the more characteristic only in not combining this with other, more observational, methods. Perhaps its most interesting finding from the viewpoint of the 1990s is women's relative liberalism regarding government intervention and control and the very large measure of general support for educative measures and not punitive ones.

The Falling Birth-Rate

Mass-Observation's 1945-published *Britain and Her Birth-Rate*[6] deals with what it terms the 'race suicide' of the falling birth-rate; that is, neither a decrease in marriage nor an increase in the age at which people marry, but the decision to have fewer children. In exploring this, Mass-Observation combined the results of a number of different kinds of investigation: 1000 interviews with married women between 20 and 45 in three different locations (London, Gloucester and 'a factory'); questions about marriage and the falling birth-rate put to Mass-Observation's National Panel; the postbag of a 'Radio Doctor' on various 'birth-rate problems'; 500 letters sent to a birth-control clinic; observation of households with children (likely to be a small number, probably those of some Mass-Observation personnel); and reports of meetings where such issues were discussed (again, likely to be meetings attended by Mass-Observation personnel). The investigation explores why such decisions were being made and what conditions might persuade women to have more children; in doing so it emphasizes that while there has been an increased use of contraception, this is an *effect*, and not a cause, of the fall in the birth-rate.

Exploring what the possible causes might be, the research found that children remained central to most women's conception of marriage, for 'it isn't marriage without them', but that women were having fewer children and also making deliberate decisions about spacing births. Their reasons centrally concerned the linked factors of money, housing, and wanting to give children the best possible chances in life – although, as the report comments, it was in fact those respondents with the most money who had fewest children. Subsidiary reasons concerned the couple's leisure, health, social attitudes, 'responsibility and selfishness', and personal make-up, and all involved women not wanting to be tied to the home in the way their mothers had been, for they 'didn't want

33

to live as their mothers had done'. The report concludes *'They are perfectly valid and good reasons, yet they mask the one real underlying motive . . . And the plain fact about the birth-rate is, in our interpretation, that women just do not want more children than they are having'.*[7]

There is a direct link here with the 1949 sex survey, for in 'Little Kinsey' too attitudes to birth control and family size are linked to 'vanguardism', that is, to women's changing views about themselves, family life and children's part in this. These two investigations together point with remarkable accuracy to the areas of 'personal life' that were to change so markedly in the 1960s and 1970s: divorce for incompatibility and an increasing divorce rate; the separation of heterosexual sexual behaviour from procreation, through better and more easily available contraception rather than a reconceptualization of 'sex'; the control of family size; an increase in levels of sexual activity prior to and outside of marriage; and an increased toleration of 'abnormal' sexual behaviour, both heterosexual and gay.

* * * * * * * *

These three Mass-Observation investigations were carried out at different times (1937–1939, 1942–1943, and 1944 respectively) in its history by different parts of the organization working from different standpoints and approaches, although the texts of each were produced by writers in its national office. All three share a concern with public sexual behaviours, or rather, in the cases of VD and the falling birth-rate, with the public manifestations and consequences of private sexual behaviours and the implications of these for public policy.[8] For many people, the Seatown/Blackpool investigation is likely to be seen as the most typically 'Mass-Observation', and its study of public attitudes to VD as a foretaste instead of the conventional 'market research' direction that the organization took in the later 1940s. Looking at the work of Mass-Observation as a whole over the period 1937–1949, however, it is actually *Britain and Her Birth-Rate*, with its complex mixing of different kinds of data woven together in an argument that adds considerable insight from the researchers/writers themselves, which is actually the most characteristic.

The three investigations produced some important findings. Mass-Observation had found that people's sexual behaviour varied a good deal in different situations, and that what was deemed morally right and proper was a product of circumstance and situation rather than an abstract code of hard-and-fast principle. It had established that a good deal of sexual behaviour actually occurred in public places, and that much of this was seen as legitimate and sanctioned, particularly regarding younger people's public conduct. It had demonstrated that people's attitudes to sexual transgression or 'abnormality' were undergoing some radical changes, such that venereal disease was in the process of becoming seen as simply a disease like any other, and that secrecy and shame were viewed as not only outmoded but also as a bar to sensible and effective treatment. And it had found that 'marriage' was itself in the process of undergoing profound changes, with deliberate reductions in family size occurring because of women's changing expectations, in particular their increasing rejection of a life bound to the home and a succession of children.

With benefit of hindsight, Mass-Observation's ability to pinpoint with accuracy key aspects of changing social behaviour is quite startlingly prescient. Mass-Observation brought to public attention aspects of the profound changes to sexual and emotional life that were to become clearly visible only in the 1960s and 1970s. It is, then, all the more to its research credit that Mass-Observation did this at the tail-end of the war period and a long while before other research bodies became aware that the changes wrought by the war would have long-term social structural as well as immediate behavioural implications. It is even more to its research credit that it insisted that such changes were linked – to put it no stronger – with the changes that women were determinedly making to their marital, maternal and sexual roles and behaviours, a point that I return to later.

Notes

1　Mark Abrams had various pre-war brushes with Harrisson, on one occasion pre-war through his discomfort at being taken north to Worktown; see Abrams (1951) *Social Surveys and Social Action* for his critique.
2　See MOA-FR 1542.
3　MOA-FR 1573; see also MOA-FR 1596 and 1599, the first and second drafts of this report minus the tables and with fewer quotations, both written in February 1943.
4　94% of men and 83% of women.
5　MOA-FR 1628.
6　Mass-Observation (1945) *Britain and Her Birth-Rate*, commissioned and published by the Advertising Standards Guild in a series concerned with 'Changes' in British society.
7　Mass-Observation (1945) *Birth-Rate* p.200.
8　Although the Blackpool research also had some implications for local authority policy and planning, as shown by the reactions of Blackpool council and various trade bodies to reports of Mass-Observation's work in the press.

Chapter 4

From *Patterns of Marriage* to *Sexual Attitudes and Lifestyles*: The Sex Survey in Context

Kinsey's *Sexual Behaviour in the Human Male* was published in 1948 and, as Tom Harrisson's Preface to 'Little Kinsey' notes, it was the direct inspiration for Mass-Observation's own sex survey. Harrisson, however, is punctilious in rejecting any idea that Mass-Observation had 'attempted to carry out a British Kinsey report': Kinsey's work covered some 12 000 men and it used 'exhaustive methods' of interviewing. Harrisson promised instead that Mass-Observation's study was 'both something less and something more than Kinsey', containing no tables but instead 'more of the actuality, the real life, the personal stuff of the problem'. For Harrisson, research results that were statistically accurate contained a 'misleading validity' that lost the human content lying behind a line-up of percentages and numbers. Nonetheless, the research was consistently known as 'Little Kinsey', and this name is apt for one particularly important reason.

Overtly Kinsey eschewed theory and promoted 'the plain facts' about the sexual behaviour of American men; implicitly, however, Kinsey's work is actually founded on a then-revolutionary set of ideas or theorization of sexual behaviour and its place within social life. There are important aspects of this 'implicit theory' in Kinsey's 1953-published *Sexual Behaviour in the Human Female*[1] as well as in his earlier study. Regardless of sexual mores or beliefs, Kinsey argued that people are actually likely to engage in a wide variety of sexual behaviour, including behaviour that public mores or beliefs present as 'abnormal' and deviant. He suggested that a researcher should assume 'everyone does everything', a stance closely related to his approach to interviewing: that when people are talked with in depth and in an open and accepting way, then they are likely to confide not only their conforming but also their supposedly deviant sexual behaviour. Relatedly, when people engage in a behaviour in large numbers, Kinsey insisted that this cannot in scientific terms be seen as abnormal or deviant. Moreover, by focusing on 'sexual behaviour in the human male' and then in 'the human female', Kinsey moved away from the more respectable 'couples and marriage' approach that characterizes many other sex surveys, those by Slater and Woodside, Chesser,

Schofield and Gorer (who are discussed later) among them. Lastly and perhaps most importantly, these aspects of Kinsey's approach are located within a framework in which sexual behaviour and sexual convention are treated as malleable, as the products of culture and history and circumstance; that is, Kinsey works within what would now be termed a 'social constructionist' approach.

Like the Kinsey Reports, Mass-Observation's 'Little Kinsey' similarly appears simply to describe numerically what different groups of informants had told its investigators, while a closer scrutiny brings to light a set of ideas that amount to a 'sexual theory', which I discuss in detail in Section Three. The British are known, or perhaps more accurately are infamous, for empirical investigations rather than for the sophistications of high theory. In the field of sex research, Britain has produced since the 1940s a kind of rogues' gallery of national sex surveys: by Eliot Slater and Moya Woodside, by Eustace Chesser, by Michael Schofield, and by Geoffrey Gorer, all working from the 1940s to the 1970s, followed between 1990 and 1994 by the Wellcome Trust's 'National Survey of Sexual Attitudes and Sexual Lifestyles'. Perhaps oddly, in view of what I earlier claimed was its pioneering importance and remarkable ability to pinpoint areas of behavioural and attitudinal change, 'Little Kinsey' does not feature importantly either in current academic or in popular accounts of sex surveys in Britain while these other surveys do.[2]

Jeffrey Weeks's history of ideas about sexuality, for instance, merely notes the Mass-Observation research as having been carried out and erroneously suggests that the first systematic study of fairly wide scope was Slater and Woodside's *Patterns of Marriage* (published in 1951). Margaret Jackson's overview of the patriarchal underpinnings of popular accounts of sex and sexuality between 1870 and 1940 does not mention Mass-Observation at all. Cate Haste's popular review of 'rules of desire' discusses the Slater and Woodside and Chesser surveys, but mentions only Mass-Observation's street sample, and this only briefly. Lesley Hall's discussion of the theory and practice of male sexuality between 1900 and 1950 refers to a wider range of material from Mass-Observation's research, concerning how sexual knowledge is gained, quack literature and men's 'on the surface' apparently greater level of sexual adjustment within marriage. However, Steve Humphries's account of the 'secret world of sex' in the first half of the century explicitly associates Mass-Observation's research with the later surveys by Slater and Woodside, Gorer and Chesser, and indeed Humphries sees Mass-Observation's work as a landmark in research concerned with the realm of the sexual.[3] In contrast, the two 1994-published books from the Wellcome Trust-funded 'National Survey of Sexual Attitudes and Lifestyles' (Johnson *et al.*, *Sexual Attitudes and Lifestyles*, and Wellings *et al.*, *Sexual Behaviour in Britain*) only briefly note the existence of unspecified 'Mass-Observation studies'. Clearly, the National Survey researchers have little idea of the scope, scale or approach of 'Little Kinsey'; indeed, in my view they are unduly dismissive of all the surveys discussed here.[4] 'Little Kinsey', with hindsight and justice, can been seen as the start of the tradition of survey-based investigation of sexual conduct in Britain[5] and I now discuss the British sex surveys that were its successors, providing a general account of each although focusing on issues concerned with gender and sexuality; as I noted earlier, my discussion of 'Little Kinsey' appears in Section Three, following the text of 'Little Kinsey' itself in Section Two.

Patterns of Marriage

Slater and Woodside's *Patterns of Marriage* was published in 1951 from research carried out between 1943 and 1946 which involved 200 soldiers and their wives, the soldiers being patients in a large London hospital. The origins of this research lay in an investigation of hereditary and familial factors in neurosis, defined as a characteristic of the men who were admitted complaining of 'inexplicable tiredness or depression, or attacks of anxiety, or . . . loss of memory',[6] rather than these being seen as responses to the war itself. On further inquiry, these men were also characterized as 'physically poor specimens' who had been nervous children in families where other members were 'unstable or neurotic', such that ordinary army life had been 'too much' for them.

It is from this sample and a control group of soldiers, also patients in the same hospital but with 'conditions that had no relation to their mental health',[7] that Slater and Woodside's account of 'patterns of marriage' is derived. In spite of labelling around half of their 330 sample members as neurotic in psychiatric terms, and also in spite of its very strong London bias, Slater and Woodside nonetheless defend the sample as permitting generalization to the whole population of Britain. First, they argue that random samples cannot eliminate all bias, and the biases of their sample are known ones. Second, they state that theirs is a good sample of an important section of the national population, the working-class Londoner. And third, they note that 'neurotics' may be so because of social factors rather than personal ones.[8]

Slater and Woodside's study covers the family background, childhood, education, occupations, sport, hobbies and sociability, and the politics, religion and values of members of the neurotic and control groups and their wives, as well as their courtship, reasons for marrying, harmony in marriage, sexual behaviour, procreation and contraception, and the effects of war on their marriages. The focus is thus upon these men's marriages and the place of sexuality within them, rather than upon sexual conduct with marriage as one of the locations of its occurence; and this marriage focus provides an important difference in emphasis from Mass-Observation's 'Little Kinsey' as well as from the Kinsey Reports themselves.

Slater and Woodside note the prevalence of 'pickups' in public places as a means by which even respectable working-class men and women meet each other, and the importance of physical but also 'mental' or emotional qualities as the basis of attraction to each other. The average working-class courtship, once in existence, is seen as simply 'settling down into' marriage after about two years, with a fairly high proportion of people having sex with their spouses – and in some cases other people as well – before marriage. The most important reasons given for marrying concerned the equation of marriage with home and happiness, with this happiness being seen as the combined product of children and being cooperative (and 'give and take', trust, 'pulling together', and 'giving in', as the basis of such cooperation).

Sex in marriage was looked at in relation to the frequency of intercourse[9] (a mode of two times a week), and Slater and Woodside note that people had an idea of an (unstated) normative standard in sexual behaviour to which people conform, with them being like others and 'just average'. However, while the men presented themselves around this 'average', their wives were both more forthcoming about their own particular situation and also expressed more negative feelings about it: sex was experienced as a duty and one that many women disliked or were bored by. Slater and Woodside note that the younger men and women had different attitudes from their elders regarding women's sexual satisfaction in marriage, seeing it as an expectation rather than something shameful. However, Slater and Woodside also point out there was considerable doubt that many of the women, including the younger women, knew what an 'orgasm' was, and thus the data on 'orgasmic frequency' is likely not to be very reliable.

Generally Slater and Woodside's sample members thought that parenthood should be the result of conscious choice, and most (4 out of every 5) had tried to space out the births of their children, although with variable success, with a similar proportion having used birth control methods at some time. Very few (*'nearly all of these men were from the Neurotic group'*[10]) wished to have no children at all: children were seen as central to marriage, a 'natural' product of it, and with a strong preference for two children, one of each sex. Having large numbers of children was firmly associated with poverty and hardship, backed by memories of long-term male unemployment and of a high proportion of the sample having themselves been a child in a large family. All of the people interviewed were aware of contraception but saw this as mechanical or chemical, rather than the withdrawal method that many of them actually used but did not term as 'contraception', with other favoured methods being condoms, Rendalls pessaries and the cap.[11] The women interviewed expressed a widespread fear of pregnancy, but remained reliant on men 'being careful' in the face of their embarrassed reluctance (or inability, given the contraceptive methods then easily available) to control their own fertility.

To a present-day reader, Slater and Woodside's research seems oddly unappreciative of the likely affects of the war itself, locating behaviours deemed neurotic within a psychoanalytic framework of understanding concerned with men's early childhood experiences rather than their adult ones. The research does recognize the change that had occurred, and was still occurring, concerning expectations of female sexual pleasure within marital relationships, and this is now perhaps one of the most interesting aspects of this study. It should also be remembered that Slater and Woodside's was the first published survey to show women's unhappiness and dissatisfaction with the sexual aspects of marriage. It retains the assumption that 'sex' is equivalent to 'intercourse', but its attention to the details of women's responses means that it also contains hints of the wider appreciation of what 'sex' might be, at least on the part of the women interviewed if not that of the researchers. However, alongside this remains the failure to explore the wide gap between the 'expectation' of pleasure and many of the wives' actual experiences of sex within marriage. The analytic problems experienced by Slater and Woodside in grappling with this issue are signalled by the related failure to explore the extent to which it was the term, or the experience, of orgasm that the women they interviewed did not understand. Slater and Woodside's data is unclear on this point, or rather, while their discussion implies it was the term, the data from the women makes it likely that for many it was indeed the experience which was not known and this is related to their more general feelings of disappointment and unhappiness.

Sexual Relationships of the English Woman

Eustace Chesser published many books and pamphlets on sexual themes between the 1940s and the 1960s; however, *The Sexual, Marital and Family Relationships of the English Woman* (1965) is probably the most important and is certainly currently the most frequently referenced of his writings.[12] *Sexual . . . Relationships of the English Woman* is an interesting study, which is less concerned with sexual or marital relations as such and more with the effects of earlier parenting and upbringing upon adult life. This survey of 10 948[13] women is not based on a single sample who were asked all of the questions on the schedule, for there were six different versions of the final questionnaire, three for single and three for married women, each of which were distributed through GPs. The length of the complete schedule was felt by Chesser and his researchers to be prohibitively long; thus its questions were distributed through the different versions, details of which are found in the book's appendices of 'specimen questionnaires'.[14] This makes interpreting the research findings extremely difficult, for picking a way through its 479 tables and 81 accompanying charts is a minefield given that it is difficult, sometimes impossible, to know exactly what part of the sample answered what questions. Moreover, although Chesser notes the biases of the sample overall (more single women than in the general population, more younger women, and more women from, in Chesser's phrase, the 'upper end of the social scale' and particularly professional and managerial groups[15]), there is no way of knowing what the characteristics of each part of the sample were and whether its biases were similar to or different from the overall ones; and obviously this too adds to the interpretational problems.

The different versions of the schedule contain perhaps surprisingly few questions on sexual behaviour as such: around 20 or so questions in each version of the questionnaire are concerned with sex,[16] and a number of these deal with the respondents' parents' sexual behaviour, or their own birth control practices, rather than their current sexual behaviour. Chesser's main concern is with sexual and more generally marital relations considered in the context of the emotional dynamics of parent/child and child/sibling relationships, the effects of parental loss, the role of parental authority and disciplining, and trends in parental control. Indeed more than half the substantive material in the book is concerned with these topics rather than with sexual relationships and feelings. While these wide interests make Chesser's study an unusual and still fascinating one,[17] they also make its results particularly difficult to come to grips with, for the interpretational issues connected with the sub-samples and the oddities of the overlapping versions of the schedule, together with the propensity to cross-tabulate every piece of information with what sometimes seems like every other, affect this data as well as that which relates more directly to sexual relations. My discussion focuses specifically on the treatment of sexual relations in Chesser's study, concerning sexual behaviour in single-adult life, within marriage, and in relation to different age cohorts.

While noting that the convention was that women especially (and men to a lesser extent) did not engage in genital sexual behaviour outside of marriage, Chesser's research shows the steady upward trend of women's involvement in a variety of sexual practices outside of marriage, including both 'petting' behaviours and heterosexual intercourse,[18] and this is the earliest explicit recognition in the British sex survey that there is more to 'sex' than the specifically genital and penetrational – 'Little Kinsey' mentions 'petting' once in an appendix, but neither mentions nor discusses it in the main text, although the various questionnaires that the text is based upon contains much information in this regard. However, although Chesser's research asks about 'petting' behaviours, this was not in any detail, and anyway analytically speaking 'petting' is treated as merely a preliminary to 'sex' itself. Moreover, the ensuing discussion of sex in adult single life makes no distinction between the younger women who were likely to marry later on, and the older women who had not married to date and were not likely to in the future, asking them all a set of questions about their 'future husbands' whether this is appropriate or not. Thus, disentangling the responses of women for whom the 'petting' and intercourse occurred before marriage and possibly with their future spouse, and those of the long-term single women, is not possible. The rest of the discussion of single adult life is similarly based on the assumption of future marriage, and contains a further set of questions about what part sexual behaviour and sexual satisfaction should have within marriage.[19]

Chesser's account of 'the married relationship' looks at levels of marital happiness, sexual satisfaction, birth control, and factors (such as temperament, education, religious conviction and so forth) that affect patterns of marital relationship, women's prior expectations of marriage, and the main factors influencing feelings of happiness and unhappiness. It is around sexual satisfaction within marriage[20] that Chesser's discussion of sexual behaviour is concentrated. While noting the general difficulties that people have in speaking about 'sexual sensations', Chesser points to a crucial change, from people feeling shame if they experienced sexual pleasure to feeling shame if they did not, a change earlier noted by Slater and Woodside particularly in relation to women. Chesser also notes that there is a reticence in admitting 'failure' in sexual terms that makes interpreting people's responses to questions about the experience of sexual pleasure or its absence extremely difficult. An additional difficulty – and one commented upon by most of the sex surveys that I discuss here – concerns what kind of language can be appropriately used by researchers that respondents will understand. Unlike Slater and Woodside, although Chesser notes the general problem he fails to consider that the terms used, and particularly that of 'orgasm', might be understood differently from the 'proper' definition assigned by the researchers or indeed not understood at all. Given this, Chesser notes the fairly large number of women who never or only infrequently experience orgasm, and also the complex relationship between orgasm and women's levels of sexual satisfaction within marriage, for, although in general the women who rarely or never experience orgasm tend to be less satisfied than women who experience orgasm always or frequently, there is nevertheless a sub-group who *are* satisfied.[21] This distinction made by women between sexual pleasure and marital happiness occurs across all of the surveys discussed here, including 'Little Kinsey', although none of them attempt to explain it as anything other than a product of women's sexual conservatism, their difference from an assumed male norm. As I noted earlier and discuss in more detail in Section Three, it was not until the advent of feminist investigations of sexual behaviour and emotion that the 'male norm' in sexual terms was displaced from the analytic centre. In the light of feminist analysis, the distinction these women make can be explained, once 'sex' is displaced from its privileged position as supposedly the most significant part of human and marital relations, as one in which they are treating sex as something specific, which they do not see, at least in the short-term, as determining their overall feelings about their marriages or their husbands.

Chesser's main analytic concern here hinges on the question of causality, in particular whether the fall in all women's levels of both orgasm and sexual satisfaction after the first few years of marriage can be causally linked with what, he claims, is a diminishment of women's physiological capacity to experience orgasm, which occurs with age.[22] Chesser ponders the question of *'whether the relationship . . . is a causal one, or whether, if so, in which direction the causality operates'*.[23] For him, the question is whether women's physiologically-determined decreasing levels of orgasm during intercourse lead to emotional and marital stress (his preferred explanation, and one that locates the source of the problem with the women), or whether it is their experientially-produced lack of orgasm that leads them to avoid having sex and thus to such stresses. The women's statements actually provide a fairly conclusive explanation, which includes their husbands ejaculating too quickly, not 'petting' enough, wanting intercourse too frequently, and being unable to express tenderness. The women locate the problem in their husbands' lack of understanding, emotional impoverishment and inept sexual practice, which results in them reducing love-making to merely 'sex' in the narrow penetrational sense.

The question of causality and in which direction it might operate is a frequent refrain in Chesser's book, and this particular section concludes with an attempt to piece together the overall factors influencing sexual satisfaction in marriage.[24] Marital happiness declines as length of marriage and age increases. However, Chesser fails to disentangle whether this includes the women who were sexually satisfied and happy earlier in their marriages as well as those who were less satisfied and less happy; and he hedges his causal bets by repeating his earlier contention that there is likely to be a physiological factor involved in the degree of sexual satisfaction/orgasm which declines with increasing age. Of course, given that Chesser's research involves women only, this is a contention about women's biological capacities, and it implies that the behaviours and feelings of their partners have little or nothing to do with their experience of orgasm or of un/happiness and stress. Thus, orgasm here is seen less as a behavioural outcome, and more as the inner and declining capacity of women.

Chesser's notable inability to extract from the great quantity of data presented any clear statements about sexual satisfactions and sexual behaviours is linked to his study's lack of a clear theoretical or conceptual framework as well as to its over-reliance on the methodological ploy of cross-tabulating everything with everything else in the hope of 'the numbers' providing such clarity. In so far as it has such a framework, this focuses on the patterning of experiences within childhood, and not on adult sexuality. Feeling swamped by its array of data and large numbers of tables and charts is a common response of readers to *Sexual . . . Relationships of the English Woman*, and most present-day commentators deal less with Chesser's lengthy discussion of sexual satisfactions, more with the dispersed mentions of cohort differences of various kinds: at different points the sample data is presented in relation to age cohorts born before 1904, between 1904 and 1914, between 1914 and 1924, between 1924 and 1934, and after 1934 (these latter would have been around 17 and under when the research was published in 1951).[25] Indeed, in methodological terms the cohort differences within the sample[26] are considerably less problematic than much of the other data, and show the occurrence of a number of interesting changes. These include: numbers of siblings decreased between the cohorts; a decline in strong parental control, but an increase in the use of physical punishment; parents becoming less likely to think sex should not be spoken about; respondents becoming more likely to speak to their girlfriends about sex and, although to a lesser extent, boyfriends also; respondents increasingly feeling that their parents had told them all they wanted to know about sex; their adherence to religious belief declining as did the strictness of its tenets; church attendance declining; pre-marital sex increasing; as did pre-marital 'petting'; the age of first menstruation falling by about a year; and an increase in respondents reading books about sex and marriage.

This cohort data provides an interesting attempt to describe and analyse change by developing a methodological instrument for doing so; that is, the age cohort groups compared against each other. The other surveys discussed here, including 'Little Kinsey', try to map change substantively, by asking their respondents about it. Thus they rely on individual opinion and assessment, and while this can yield interesting results – in my view most convincingly so in the case of 'Little Kinsey' – it is Chesser's approach that provides a more focused and precise measure which can compare a number of different groups across a lengthy period of time. It is then all the more disappointing that so little of the cohort data is concerned with sexual behaviours and relations as such and that the age cohort data was used only tangentially in Chesser's study. All of these surveys are concerned with change, sexual change specifically, and I return later to the methodological and other issues involved.

Slater and Woodside's psychoanalytically-influenced approach leads them into a narrow reductionism of behaviour, while, interestingly, Chesser's utilization of psychoanalytic ideas leads him to explore in considerable depth a wide variety of parenting behaviour and the responses to it by 'former children'. Although his research has a relational focus signalled in its title as well as its concern with parent/child dynamics, Chesser's analysis assigns significance only to past relationships and not present ones. It is this that leads to the very clear data on women's sexual dissatisfactions within marriage being 'explained' by actually being explained away through essentialist ideas about biology and ageing rather than by reference to the marital relationship itself. It is almost as though at the very 'moment', analytically speaking, that Chesser approached the crux of the problem that his research, as well as that of Slater and Woodside and 'Little Kinsey', had identified, he shied away from the explanation of 'causality' that his data provides in the shape of the very clear analysis provided by the women respondents. The emphasis on 'the past' that is so central to Chesser's Freudian approach unfortunately prevented him from seeing what was under his analytic nose.

Sexual Behaviour of Young People

Michael Schofield's *The Sexual Behaviour of Young People*[27] came out of an international conference on venereal disease, at which discussion of 'promiscuity' led to more general discussion of sexual behaviour among young people as the possible cause of increased rates of VD, particularly gonorrhoea. The lack of adequate statistics for a representative group of young people led to Nuffield funding this research, which investigates the sexual attitudes and behaviour of young people. In Schofield's research, a large random sample of young people aged between 15 and 19 was interviewed about family background and leisure activities as well as sexual attitudes and behaviour. Special techniques were adopted to ensure that 'the truth' was obtained: an ordinary market-research interview approach was eschewed in favour of training interviewers *'so that they might learn how to win the confidence of the young people in a short time'*;[28] the questions were piloted through discussion with groups of teenagers; the interviewers were all young and interviewed teenagers of the same sex as themselves; and there were six call-back visits before an interview was abandoned.[29] A total of 1873 interviews were carried out; and Schofield emphasizes that no comparison of the results with other research is possible because of the absence of other representative random research.

For the majority of the young people questioned, their first heterosexual sexual contact came with kissing on a first date. However, often this was not open-mouthed 'French kissing' even for those who already had prior sexual experience. Thereafter, a variety of eight 'petting' activities short of heterosexual penetrative sex might occur: for many, however, penetrative sex was not engaged in, although, of those who did, more of them were boys than girls. When penetrative sex occurred for the first time, it was unpremeditated for over four-fifths of both girls and boys; it 'just happened'. Schofield also notes that over a fifth of the boys knew of homosexual behaviour among their schoolfriends and one in 20 were involved in such behaviour themselves, while over a tenth of the girls knew of schoolfriends and one in 40 were involved themselves; and he suggests that this is liable to be an underestimate in both cases.

When heterosexual sexual intercourse occurred, more girls than boys associated it with feelings of love, and more boys than girls with feelings of desire, but there was a large number of both sexes for whom the primary feeling was rather one of curiosity. Moreover, when intercourse first occurred, for half of the boys and for two-thirds of the girls it was neither a successful nor a very pleasurable experience, with many saying how disenchanted they felt.[30] Interestingly, these feelings occur alongside the fact that over four-fifths of the boys and nearly a third of the girls nonetheless report themselves having reached a 'climax', in the term Schofield used. For most of these young people, penetrative sex took place out of a sexual learning process, of moving through different kinds of physical/sexual intimacies. Schofield, like Chesser, calls this lengthy and complex process involving a large number of different although related behaviours by the term 'petting' and then differentiates it from 'sex', i.e. intercourse. 'Sex' in this sense occurred by and large when they were over the age of 16 – by the age of 15 only about one in twenty of the boys and one in fifty of the girls had had this experience. When it occurred, for about half of the boys and two-thirds of the girls, their first partner was older than them and, typically, was someone already known to them who was likcly thereafter to become a steady partner.

The average age that the young people 'found out about sex' was about 12 years, with boys usually finding out from friends, and girls from a combination of friends and their mothers. A minority[31] had received information about sex from teachers, but this occurred only at age 14 or later. Schofield notes class differences here, with middle-class children 'finding out' at an earlier age, middle-class girls earliest of all. And for around two-thirds of the boys and a third of the girls, their parents had said nothing at all to them about sex.

Contraception was known about by a large majority of both the boys and the girls. Of the sexually active group of these young people, nearly a half said they used some form (unspecified) of birth control, while a quarter said they never did (and a third of these boys 'didn't care' about this[32]). Most of the sexually active girls neither took contraceptive precautions themselves nor insisted that their partners did – and of course it has to be remembered that when this research was carried out the pill was not available to the vast majority of these young women.

In relation to venereal disease, which provided the rationale for funding Schofield's research, a significant minority of both boys and girls knew nothing about it at all, while a third of the sample could describe no symptoms. Only four of the boys and two of the girls had been to a clinic suspecting that they might have a venereal disease, with two boys and one girl having an infection confirmed, figures which hardly support the high level of public concern that had initiated this research.

Overall, the majority of both boys and girls in this sample of young people were highly family-centred and wanted marriage and children for themselves, although a quarter of them wanted a 'good time' beforehand because they saw life after marriage as dreary. The main differences between the boys and the girls were, first, that the girls wanted to marry at an earlier age than the boys, for many of them before they were 21; and, second, that although the boys wanted to have sex, they were morally critical of the girls who were their sexual partners.

Schofield's research looks in more detail at what 'sex' consists of than either Slater and Woodside or Chesser, in particular because the various behavioural components or stages of 'petting' are looked at as these young people's route to heterosexual intercourse. This research proposes that more 'sex' is being engaged in by then-contemporary young people than before. However, by treating the 'early starters' as somehow odd or deviant, Schofield fails to recognize that his research shows that for the large majority of these young people their sexual relationships are subject to the same kinds of codes and controls as the courtship behaviour (not always accurately seen as non-sexual) of earlier generations. From the viewpoint of the 1990s, two of the most interesting aspects of Schofield's research are the noted, but not investigated, occurrence of homosexual sexual behaviour, and the, at least initial, lack of sexual pleasure reported by both sexes. Given both the levels of reporting homosexual behaviour and Schofield's view that this is likely to be an underestimate, the exclusively heterosexual focus of this study is perhaps surprising, and it is I think related to the then-perceived outrageousness of asking young people about their sexual behaviour in a non-condemnatory way rather than any lack of awareness or interest on Schofield's part.[33] In relation to young people's lack of reported sexual pleasure on initial intercourse, the social constructionist approach sees not only understandings of what 'sex' is, but also how pleasure is defined and attached to particular behaviours, as the product of social factors. Given the great western cultural emphasis relating sexual pleasure to penetration, particularly for boys, their *reporting* the absence of such pleasure, as well as the absence itself, is interesting and noteworthy but unfortunately is not explored in any detail. It has been largely because of feminist thinking that such assumptions about the supposedly exclusively penetrational nature of male sexual feelings have been problematized within research, although in the main it is adult rather than adolescent male sexuality that it has focused upon.

Sex and Marriage in England

Geoffrey Gorer's *Exploring English Character*,[34] published in 1955, used over 10 000 questionnaires sent in response to a newspaper discussion of 'English character' to produce a representative sample of some 5000. These questionnaires were analysed using the same new computerized methods that had six years earlier excited Mass-Observation's researchers into applying them to the sex research that became 'Little Kinsey'. A number of questions in this study were concerned with marital and sexual matters; and from these Gorer concluded that the English viewed marriage with great seriousness as the central emotional 'falling in love' experience of their lives, for even those who favoured sex before marriage did so because they saw it as a means of avoiding sexual ignorance and maladjustment in marriage. Then, in the late 1960s, Gorer obtained funding from another newspaper, the *Sunday Times*, to restudy those aspects of his earlier research concerned with sexual behaviour.

Gorer's 1971-published *Sex and Marriage in England Today*[35] repeated the 1950s questions on attitudes to sex and marriage, but also included many new ones on individual sexual behaviour. His sample was of 949 men and 1037 women aged 16–45, from a mixture of conurbations and different sized towns; and it under-represents the separated and divorced in the sampled age groups,[36] although discussion of the results focuses specifically on the married rather than the single. Gorer's *Exploring English Character* had noted that, of those who were 'not interested in sex', '*quite a number volunteered the statement they were homosexual*'.[37] However, these people are not mentioned again; while his later *Sex and Marriage* never mentions homosexuality except in a very brief discussion of attitudes to it, rather than 'it', homosexuality itself.[38] Indeed, unlike Schofield, but like the other sex surveys before the Wellcome National Survey, Gorer's *Sex and Marriage* asks no detailed questions about what sample members do when they 'have sex', which results both in all the many behaviours and complications of sexual and emotional relations being glossed under the one term 'sex', and in the related implication that sex and intercourse are synonymous. My discussion focuses on the emphasis in Gorer's 1971 research on sexual behaviour rather than sexual attitudes, and on the 'sexual double standard' that his work discerns.

Over a quarter of the married men and nearly two-thirds of the married women said they had been virgins at marriage, and an additional fifth of the men and quarter of the women said that the person they later married was the first person they had had sex with. Although a higher proportion of men than women had had sex before the age of 17, by the age of 24 a higher proportion of women had done so,[39] with working-class people in general becoming sexually active at a younger age than the middle class. Gorer notes one change particularly between his two studies, that by 1971 more women were having sex before marriage, although he concludes there was still a 'sexual double standard' existing between women and men, to an extent regarding behaviour, even more so regarding attitudes, with the main influence here being religion rather than class or education. Fewer women in the first than in the second study thought that sex in marriage was very im- portant, while by the time of *Sex and Marriage* men and women more or less equally stated its importance, and Gorer interprets this as a shift by women in the direction of greater sexual liberation. However, it is at least equally likely that it is a product of the difference between behaviour and attitude that Gorer notes (and which is central to 'Little Kinsey's' approach), an artefact of the construction of his schedule, with women in greater numbers verbally simply going along with this orthodoxy in one part of the survey but then reporting different behaviour in another.

Gorer notes a close convergence between the rates of sexual intercourse claimed by men and by women, even when responses are broken down for the married and the unmarried.[40] Regarding enjoyment of intercourse, little change between Gorer's two surveys was discerned, with men still emphasizing physical enjoyment more than women; and although by 1971 more younger people stressed its physical enjoyment, this was predominantly younger men, not women. Gorer considers this as further evidence of the sexual double standard, although it is equally legitimately interpreted as a statement of fact by women, as is the sexual difference Gorer notes in the level of experience of orgasm. The word 'orgasm' was not used in the main research, as in the pilot it was understood by few of the sample members, and so 'a real physical climax . . . in the same way as men' was used instead.[41] Relatedly, a tenth of the men but a quarter of the women reported not having orgasms at all; again, Gorer sees this as more evidence of a sexual double standard, although it too can be seen as a statement of fact, and indeed evidence from other sex research, such as Kinsey or Masters and Johnson, suggests this is precisely how it should be interpreted.

When discussing unfaithfulness, Gorer notes those who did not think husbands should necessarily be faithful and the slightly smaller number who did not think that wives should necessarily be so,[42] and he suggests that the disproportionate number of women thinking this about husbands provides yet more evidence of a sexual double standard (rather than, for example, merely a recognition of the realities of adultery). He also notes that women condemn casual affairs more than men, but do so equally regarding the women and men who engage in them, and also that women think that adultery resulted from men being over-sexed (perhaps reflecting the rationale often used by adulterous men to justify their behaviour), while men think it a natural thing to do as long as the doer can get away with it.

Although Gorer's research contains a very large amount of tabular data, by and large it avoids the analytic problems that I have noted with Chesser's work. This is in part because Gorer uses each chapter to present a narrative concerned with a particular topic rather than assuming that a large amount of data will somehow 'speak for itself', but it is also because his main analytic concern is with the 'sexual double standard'. This gives Gorer's research a greater readability than Chesser's, even though it too contains a large number of tables; its analytic focus also gives it a much more contemporary 'feel' than Chesser's relentless empiricism. As I have suggested, the data that comprises Gorer's 'double standard' can at each point be interpreted differently. Nonetheless it is important to note that his research does at least recognize that there are differences between women's and men's experiences of and opinions about sex within and outside marriage, and it also emphasizes that such difference requires both recognition and explanation.

Sexual Attitudes and Lifestyles

After a troubled early history in which AIDS politicking led Downing Street to require that previously agreed funding arrangements should be withdrawn,[43] the 'National Survey of Sexual Attitudes and Lifestyles' was funded by the Wellcome Trust and interviewing started in 1990, pilot research having been carried out earlier. The two books from this research, Johnson *et al.*'s *Sexual Attitudes and Lifestyles*, and Wellings *et al.*'s *Sexual Behaviour in Britain*, were preceded by articles concerned with the research's methodological underpinnings, procedures and its approach to the interpretation of findings, as well as reports of its initial substantive findings.[44]

The objectives of the National Survey are located firmly within concern about HIV and AIDS considered in an epidemiological tradition, not a broader social science one,[45] in which the production of reliable data about sexual practices across countries is seen as a means of understanding the differential spread of HIV world-wide.[46] This research was carried out to provide 'baseline' information on the sexual behaviour of the general population, so increasing understanding of variations in such behaviour, and thereby allowing mathematical modelling techniques to be used in predicting transmission of the HIV virus, while also looking at such behaviour in the context of health education planning and services.[47] Perhaps over-confidently in the light of 'Little Kinsey' and the other post-war sex surveys discussed here, the National Survey researchers claim that '*Sexual behaviour is one of the few remaining areas of human conduct uncharted by random sample survey research*'.[48] Their sample was of 18 876 people and, as compared with the 1981 Census and the 1985 General Household Survey, is seen as representative of the demographic structure of the population of Great Britain, including the proportions of those living in cities, towns and rural areas. In addition to the main interview, the more 'sensitive' questions on sexual practices and other high-risk behaviours were asked in a self-completion booklet.

Various methodological procedures were adopted to ensure that interviewing would be neither intrusive nor invade privacy and that the results would be reliable and valid in statistical terms.[49] A prime concern of the National Survey lies with issues of representativeness and comparability, which is seen as largely the product of technical considerations concerning the structure of the *sample*; and thus the detailed information given about the achieved sample and the stress on problems with quota-based random samples, and use of what is seen as a less problematic 'probability sample' using the 'Kish grid' of household composition and fixed interview choice in this research. Validity is discussed in the context of the quality of data the sample provided and around problems with memory recall rather than dishonesty or deliberate misrepresentation. It is also dealt with in relation to issues of precision and reliability, primarily by emphasizing the *robustness of responses* – that is, the consistency of what is said between test and re-test, between interview and self-completions, and by comparison with other nationally available statistics (such as those on abortion or attendance at STD clinics). The conduct of the survey *interview* is also seen to be involved here; it started with less personal and more general questions, and this is seen to facilitate a feeling of trust between interviewer and respondent. Questions were carefully phrased using a neutral interviewing style, a public semi-formal language and the written provision to respondents of key terms and phrases. More sensitive questions in the interview were asked by means of lists on show cards so that answers could be pointed to or said in the form of numbers or letters; and as already noted, the most sensitive questions of all were contained in self-completion booklets, concerning sexual practices, numbers of heterosexual and homosexual sexual partners, drug injection and STD clinic attendance.[50] Respondents were assured of confidentiality and anonymity; and their honesty is seen to be assured by the neutral and non-judgmental phrasing of questions, a 'permissive' interviewing style, and the assurance of confidentiality.

To date the most contentious aspect of the National Survey's substantive results concerns its claims about the incidence of male homosexuality.[51] Sample members were asked in the self-completion questions about any sexual experience of any kind with same-sex as well as opposite-sex partners.

'*Questions ranged from same gender sexual experience as defined by the respondent, through experience involving genital contact of different kinds, to reporting of homosexual partners*', with the researchers concluding that '*the "prevalence" of homosexual experience depends on the definition of what constitutes such an experience and over what time period it is measured*'.[52] The conclusion is that only a small percentage of the male population in Britain as a whole – just over 1% – are currently involved with a same-sex partner, although there are significantly larger numbers of men with current same-sex partnerships in London – around 3.5% – compared with Great Britain as a whole, a difference that is explained as the product of the migration of gay men to London from other parts of Britain.[53]

These claims have been contentious for a number of important reasons connected with the National Survey's methodological approach and assumptions, with critics suggesting that the figures are a gross under-representation of gay male sexual behaviour.[54] The National Survey's researchers do note that the results of surveys of any '*socially censured behaviours have to be regarded as minima*', but at the same time they also emphasize that their results are consistent with French and American research and that '*The research instrument itself . . . can be applied to other population subgroups to obtain comparable data*'.[55] However, they fail to take sufficiently into account that their methodological approach is not one best suited to encourage people to disclose any taboo or stigmatized sexual experience, particularly considering that problems concerning gay self-disclosure have been central to discussion of the problematics of 'coming out', especially so regarding disclosure of sexual orientation outside of gay sub-cultural contexts.[56] That is, for many, probably still most, gay people, central to self-perception of being gay is precisely an absence of self-disclosure except in certain highly specific and safe social contexts and with only very particular persons, while the National Survey makes the assumption that a two-hour interview with a stranger will successfully enable such consequential self-disclosure, an incredible failure to grasp the personal and political dynamics involved.[57]

In fact, it is more likely that only those gay people who have sub-cultural supports (for example, in London, Manchester or other large cities that offer both anonymity and a large gay community), and/or those who reject conventional stigmatized views of behaving and being gay and take a highly politicized stance regarding gay self-disclosure, would be likely to respond 'honestly' to questions posed within this research. Thus, Project Sigma, a research project funded under AIDS Initiative funding, carried out an earlier study asking nearly 500 gay men whether they would take part in the Wellcome study if approached. Half said they would refuse, and a further third said they would participate but hide the fact they were gay. In a useful and sensible article discussing this and related problems with the National Survey, Peter Keogh makes three important criticisms.[58] First, the National Survey's refusal rate – around 31.1% of the planned interviews[59] – is likely to be the key to understanding the low proportion of gay respondents, along with the probability that a significant number of respondents hid (i.e. lied about) their sexuality. Second, the schedule asks about heterosexual and gay experience in different ways, through 'leading' questions ('when did you last . . .') regarding the former and 'prohibitive' ones ('have you ever . . .') regarding the latter, thus effectively discouraging openness about gay experiences. Third, the order of questions asks about heterosexuality first, and then about homosexuality, thereby privileging the former – and, although not mentioned by Keogh, this also sets up an opposition between them as two separate 'lifestyles' when for many people such behaviour is likely to overlap in complex ways.

In addition, if the National Survey under-represents the gay male experience, then it does this in spades for lesbian women. Only 0.3% of the total sample, for example, are described as having lesbian sexual experience in the terms used by the National Survey. Also, there is a constant slide in writings by the National Survey researchers, often within a single sentence, from 'gay people' to 'gay men', which indicates either a disabling level of discomfort with lesbianism and/or a lack of interest in women's sexual experiences compared with those of men. Effectively, lesbianism does not figure on the sexual map in any significant way at all, and nor is this 'absence' seen, as surely it should be, as a factual problem, the existence of which needs to be demonstrated, discussed and explained. This seems to be the product of a more general lack of interest in women's sexuality and sexual experiences, whether heterosexual or gay. One demonstration of this comes through the National Survey focus on only those behaviours deemed to be 'high risk' in relation to HIV/AIDS: genital or anal, penetrational or otherwise, involving the exchange of body fluids. This leads to an overly narrow and one-dimensional construction and discussion of heterosexuality as much as homosexuality. Thus, extraordinarily, it is the *vagina* that the National Survey researchers define as women's 'sexual organs' in the same way that the penis is men's, thus '*Genital area a man's penis or a woman's vagina – that is, the sex organs*';[60] that is, that bit of women's anatomy which is the 'site' of the high-risk exchange of bodily fluids. The clitoris is not mentioned, let alone 'defined', anywhere in this research and nor is the occurence or absence of orgasm or sexual pleasure more widely in either women or men. Desire and pleasure are absent, along with consent and force, lust and pain, sorrow and joy. The interpretational concern throughout is whether sexual behaviour is 'high risk', and not whether it involves constraint or force, passion or pleasure. There is a lack of interest in the meaning of sexual behaviour for the respondents, regardless of whether this is mediated by passion or rape, desire or fear; indeed, meaning is specifically and deliberately omitted from this research as outside of its concerns.[61] Thereby almost everything that is analytically interesting and behaviourally consequential about sexual practices, indeed that would explain the occurence of such practices, is excluded from the National Survey. There are numbers and percentages aplenty, but little awareness that what gives life to these is how people understand and feel about what they do and do not do; research that excludes this, in my view, will not be able to explain very much of anything.

I shall return to the National Survey in the context of my discussion of the Hite surveys. However, it is instructive to note here that its remarks about the low incidence of lesbian sexual behaviour are based on a sample of only *31 women*. This is a smaller number than the circle of my own lesbian friends and acquaintances, but because of its claimed 'representativeness' as 0.3% of the entire sample it is supposedly a better basis on which to make knowledge-claims about the existence of lesbianism as a 'life style', as well as, more trivi-ally, lesbian sexual experience.

The National Survey's epidemiological concerns also give it a curiously old-fashioned methodological stance, for there is no awareness that its 'facts' and 'findings' in the form of its numbers and percentages might be artefac-tual to structural aspects of this particular survey. Two important factors here concern ethnicity and literacy. Various examples of the sexual 'definitions' inquired about are provided in the National Survey's self-completion book-let, and, as already noted, questions about the more 'difficult' areas of sexu-al behaviour are in this booklet also. There is a brief mention of refusal at the self-completion stage of the interview, although this is not linked with possi-ble literacy issues,[62] nor is there any acknowledgement of the high levels of reading and writing problems found by other research (typically around 15% of the population, and particularly high among first generation immigrants). There is no discussion of the likely impact of this on any survey, like this one, so dependent on its self-completion element. Moreover, this problem will have been compounded by, not only the self-completion booklet, but the whole survey, having been carried out in English only; some people in the UK's many ethnic communities will be literate only in a first language that is not English, and of course others in neither, while particularly older people may also have problems with spoken English beyond the very basic.[63] These are neither minor nor insignificant issues, but central and crucial to any research that claims representativeness, affecting as they do upwards of a fifth of the total population. However, there are no signs that these issues were taken seriously within this research: there is no discussion, for example, about whether the schedule and self-completions should have been in more than one language, nor whether interviewers with a range of first-languages should have been used, nor with the general issue of literacy in relation to the use of the self-completion booklets.

Notes

1 Alfred Kinsey (1953) *Sexual Behaviour in the Human Female*.
2 See Jeffrey Weeks (1981/1989) *Sex, Politics and Society*; Steve Humphries (1988) *A Secret World of Sex*; Richard Davenport-Hines (1990) *Sex, Death and Punishment*; Lesley Hall (1991) *Hidden Anxieties: Male Sexuality, 1900–1950*; Cate Haste (1992) *Rules of Desire*; Margaret Jackson (1994) *The Real Facts of Life*; Anne Johnson *et al.* (1994) *Sexual Attitudes and Lifestyles*; and Kaye

Wellings *et al.* (1994) *Sexual Behaviour in Britain*.

3 Steve Humphries (1988) *World of Sex* pp.40–42.

4 Johnson *et al.* (1994) *Sexual Attitudes* pp.3–5, Wellings *et al.* (1994) *Sexual Behaviour* pp.3–4.

5 'Little Kinsey' was only vaguely known about by most of its successors; however, Eustace Chesser not only knew about it, but offered to write up the research for book publication, and he clearly recognized its importance for the serious investigation of sexual conduct in Britain.

6 Eliot Slater and Moira Woodside (1951) *Patterns of Marriage*, p.8.

7 Slater and Woodside (1951) *Patterns of Marriage* p.12.

8 Slater and Woodside (1951) *Patterns of Marriage* p.29; that is, they retain the notion of neuroticism, accept that its origins may be found in social factors, but only those experienced within childhood and not also in adult life.

9 There are interesting issues in interpreting this term, for respondents may well have used it to encompass a wider set of sexual behaviours than the researchers seemingly intended by their usage of the term; see also Chapter 2, note 21.

10 Slater and Woodside (1951) *Patterns of Marriage* p.178.

11 Slater and Woodside (1951) *Patterns of Marriage* p.294.

12 See Eustace Chesser (1941, 1946, 1949a, 1949b, 1965); and Chesser and Dawe (1946); Chesser *et al.* (1961); *The Sexual, Marital and Family Relationships of the English Woman* is Chesser (1965).

13 Chesser nowhere states the total number. This has been calculated (by Stanley) from the figures in *Sexual . . . Relationships* p.13, concerned with the geographical distribution of sample members.

14 These are 82, 67, 93, 69, 91 and 60 questions in length respectively.

15 However, it needs to be noted that only the single women's own class/occupational position is known, for Chesser gauges the married women's exclusively through that of their husbands (see *Sexual . . . Relationships* pp.17–18).

16 This is explicitly defined as genital, penetrational and heterosexual.

17 For instance, Chesser's data on cohort changes in patterns of parental control and the relationship between this and the changing incidence of physical punishment of children is particularly interesting, and offers insights as yet unexplored in current research concerned with re/constructions of the notion of 'childhood'.

18 'Petting' is defined as 'a hetero-sexual relationship other than sexual intercourse' on p.329 of *Sexual . . . Relationships*; changes in the incidence of intercourse and 'petting' are discussed on pp.329–334.

19 See Chesser (1965) *Sexual . . . Relationships* pp.376–391.

20 Chesser (1965) *Sexual . . . Relationships* pp.421–454.

21 See here the discussion in Chesser (1965) *Sexual . . . Relationships* pp.422–424.

22 Chesser (1965) *Sexual . . . Relationships* p.426.

23 Chesser (1965) *Sexual . . . Relationships* p.439.

24 See for example Chesser (1965) *Sexual . . . Relationships* pp. 439, 446 and 449, as well as pp.452–4.

25 See Chesser's Table 276 and Table 277, *Sexual . . . Relationships* pp.311, 313; and also the later discussion therein of the cohort element in this study.

26 My discussion of these below encompasses the cohort tables and discussions on pp.58, 99, 100-1, 163, 165, 167, 236–8, 239–40, 311, 318 and 496 of *Sexual . . . Relationships*.

27 Michael Schofield (1965 and 1968) *The Sexual Behaviour of Young People*. All

references are to this Penguin edition.

28 Schofield *Sex . . . Young People* p.21.

29 See Schofield *Sex . . . Young People* pp.33–35, 239–45 and 246–54 for discussions of method.

30 And for 28% of the boys and 39% of the girls these feelings persisted even after this first experience, although Schofield's interview schedule contains no means of exploring why this lack of pleasure occurred or persisted.

31 Around 12% of boys and 18% of girls.

32 Schofield *Sex . . . Young People* p.92.

33 His later work included a book (Schofield, 1976) on *Promiscuity*.

34 Geoffrey Gorer (1955) *Exploring English Character*.

35 Geoffrey Gorer (1971) *Sex and Marriage in England Today*.

36 The sample consisted of 28% single men, 70% married, 1% divorced and 1% separated; and of 11% single women, 86% married, 1% divorced and 1% separated.

37 Gorer (1971) *Sex and Marriage* p.80.

38 Gorer (1971) *Sex and Marriage* pp.242-63.

39 By age 17, 16% compared with 5%; and by age 24, 67% compared with 65%.

40 Those claiming that intercourse occurred three times a week or more represented 24% of the married and 20% overall of the sexually active; those claiming that intercourse occurred once or twice a week represented 36% of the married and 39% overall of the sexually active; and those claiming that intercourse occurred once a week or less represented 37% of the married and 30% overall of the sexually active.

41 Gorer (1971) *Sex and Marriage* p.161.

42 10% and 7% respectively.

43 Joint Centre for Survey Methods Newsletter (1989); and also Wellings *et al.* (1990) 'Sexual lifestyles under scrutiny'.

44 Field and Wadsworth (1989) 'Developing the methodology for a national survey of sexual attitudes and lifestyles'; Wellings *et al.* (1990) 'Sexual lifestyles'; Wadsworth and Johnson (1991) 'Measuring sexual behaviour'; and also Johnson *et al.* (1992) 'Sexual lifestyles and HIV risk'.

45 Field and Wadsworth (1989) 'Developing the methodology' p.6; Wadsworth and Johnson (1991) 'Measuring sexual behaviour' p.367; Johnson *et al.* (1992) 'Sexual lifestyles and HIV risks' p.410.

46 Wadsworth and Johnson (1991) 'Measuring sexual behaviour' p.367.

47 Field and Wadsworth (1989) 'Developing the methodology'.

48 Wadsworth and Johnson (1991) 'Measuring sexual behaviour' p.367.

49 Wellings *et al.* (1990) 'Sexual lifestyles under scrutiny'; and Wadsworth and Johnson (1991) 'Measuring sexual behaviour'.

50 See here Johnson *et al.* (1994) *Sexual Attitudes and Lifestyles* pp.345–422, where all the schedule questions and those in the self-completion booklets are provided.

51 It confines its discussion to gay men rather than also including lesbian women, and this is presumably linked to the perception of those most at risk to HIV infection; thus also the questions on STD clinic attendance and drug injection along with male homosexual 'contact' in the self-completion booklet.

52 Johnson *et al.* (1992) 'Sexual lifestyles and HIV risk' p.411.

53 The figures regarding same-sex male partnerships are: 6.1% of men in Great Britain as a whole have had some level of homosexual experience, while 3.6%

have had a same-sex partner at some point in their lives, 1.4% have had one in the past five years, and 1.1% have done so in the past year. In London 11.9% of men have had some level of homosexual experience, 8.6% have had a same-sex partner at some point in their lives, 4.6% have had one in the past five years, and 3.5% in the past year. See here Johnson *et al.* (1992) 'Sexual lifestyles and HIV risk' p.411, and also Johnson *et al.* (1994) Sexual Attitudes and Lifestyles pp.183–224 and Wellings *et al.* (1994) *Sexual Behaviour in Britain* pp.178–229.

54 See, for example, the front-page story headed 'Research team defends 1-in-90 gay sex claim' in *The Independent on Sunday*, 23 January 1994, p.1, which outlines criticisms of this aspect of the research from gay groups and researchers and its defence by Anne Johnson and Kaye Wellings, two of the researchers involved.

55 However, there are studies other than the surveys quoted by the National Survey reports that have found very much higher percentages. The surveys referenced adopt a very similar kind of approach to that adopted by the National Survey itself: 'findings' are significantly affected by research design, in particular the survey assumption that people will 'tell all', as I discuss in this section. See here Johnson *et al.* (1992) 'Sexual lifestyles and HIV risk' p.412.

56 A classic lesbian feminist text here is Julia Penelope and Susan Wolfe (Eds) (1980 and 1989) *The Original Coming Out Stories*. For the British context, see Suzanne Neild and Rosalind Pearson (Eds) (1992) *Women Like Us*; Hall Carpenter Archives (1989a) *Inventing Ourselves* and (1989b) *Walking After Midnight*; and Brighton Ourstory Project (1992) *Daring Hearts: Lesbian and Gay Lives of 50s and 60s*.

57 The National Survey used interviews in order to produce numbers – but in a very different way from Kinsey. Kinsey stayed in a local area speaking at groups and organizations about his research, then talking informally and in an open-ended way with people in social contexts rather than that of a formal interview, and over many hours and sometimes successive days, with no fixed list of formalized questions. The National Survey research was carried out in one formal interview with a fixed list of formalized questions lasting at most two hours and with no prior or subsequent social interaction between interviewer and interviewee. I discuss Kinsey's interviewing approach again in Section Three.

58 Peter Keogh 'Swelling the numbers' *The Pink Paper* 4 February 1994, p.13; see also the useful discussion in Peter Tatchell (1993) 'Where are this missing millions?' and also the letter to the editor 'Chaps were telling porkies' on p.30 of the same issue of *Gay Times*.

59 Johnson *et al.* (1994) pp.46–49. I have derived this percentage from adding together the 5.9% who refused to give the information needed to allow an interviewee to be selected from household members, and the 25.2% who refused to participate (p.46). In my view the response rate of 63.3%, and the related refusal rate, is explained away through caveats as actually 'comparing favourably' with previous – unreferenced – British studies of sexual behaviour (see here pp.48–9). There is no discussion of the likely reasons for such a refusal rate or of its possible impact on the achieved results.

60 See Johnson *et al.* 1994, p. 349 and also p. 369.

61 Johnson *et al.* (1994) p. 8.

62 'However, despite a careful introduction to the self-completion booklet, 3.7% of men and 4.0% of women failed to complete it' Johnson *et al.* (1994) p.57.

63 As Director of the Manchester Rochdale 'Social Change and Economic Life'
    Initiative surveys (a random, Kish-grid based, survey of 1000 people, and a re-
    lated household survey of 300 of these people and, where they had them, their
    partners), in call-back doorstep interviews following the second 'household' sur-
    vey it was found that issues concerned with ethnicity and language affected a
    large number of people, for the local population included Italians, Poles,
    Ukrainians and Latvians as well as people whose families were of New
    Commonwealth origin, and literacy issues also affected a large number of indige-
    nous white English. The combined effects involved nearer 20% than 15% of
    those interviewed.

Chapter 5

Theorizing While Appearing Not To? Ideas and the British Sex Survey

In looking at the research context of which 'Little Kinsey' was a part, I have concentrated on discussing the British tradition of large-scale random sample-based surveys of sexual attitudes and sexual behaviours conducted in the period after 'Little Kinsey' was carried out. However, these surveys were by no means the only public pronouncements of 'the facts' about sex through this period.[1] From the 1940s on, Royal Commissions, popular textbooks, newspaper, magazine and radio discussions, have dealt with sex education, the birth-rate, venereal disease, promiscuity, adultery, teenage sexuality, women's sexual 'problems', and more.[2] In addition, a wide range of other kinds of research-based investigations of sexual conduct have been carried out, smaller-scale studies including ethnographic research on sex and social structure, laboratory investigations of physiological 'sexual response', and, latterly, interview studies of sexual beliefs and practices. Also, a very large number of 'popular' surveys have been sponsored and published by newspapers and magazines and a smaller number of academic surveys of particular sub-sections of the population have been carried out. Thus, the random sample survey tradition discussed here represents only one, albeit important, strand within a wider, immensely complex and often contradictory public discourse about 'the sexual' in all its aspects.

Like Kinsey, and also like Mass-Observation's 'Little Kinsey', the British sex surveys that I have discussed are apparently entirely empirical and descriptive in approach, but they actually articulate a coherent set of ideas about sexuality and its relationship to other aspects of social life. It is these ideas, which link together to provide a framework of understanding, that I now discuss. There are, as I have already noted, differences of approach and emphasis between these surveys. Nonetheless, their ideas content shares a number of distinctive features, and these bring them considerably closer to the views and understandings of the people who were the objects of these researches than the authors would have been eager to recognize. In particular, and with the apparent exception of the National Survey, such surveys operate in a context characterized by the taken-for-grantedness of what 'sex' is: everyone is assumed to know and agree about the 'what', 'when' and 'who' of sex, to the extent that the basic behaviours with which these surveys are concerned are not looked at in any detail. The gloss of 'sex' as 'intercourse' is more often than not used as though there can be no variant behaviour involved beneath this visible and easily investigated tip. This is linked to the additional assumption that 'what people do' is governed, indeed determined, by 'the natural', by some kind of innate biological urge or imperative that is universally experienced and enacted. However, it is clear from the various 'problems' discussed by these studies that what was considered to be 'natural' underwent some fairly wide-reaching changes over the half-century between the 1940s and the 1990s, and also that such changes impinged considerably on the research carried out.

Thus, Slater and Woodside note that younger women compared with older women not only expected more of marriage but tended to relate marital problems to difficult material circumstances; and they also note that the women interviewed frequently had no idea of what was meant by 'an orgasm', and were perhaps equally uncomprehending of some of the other terms used. Similarly, while Eustace Chesser fails to look in any detail at what 'intercourse' and 'petting' consist of, his research does pinpoint the changes that had occurred regarding women's increased sexual experience both before and outside marriage. Michael Schofield's investigation of young people's sexual behaviour begins to deconstruct the monolith of 'sex', looking at a range of constituent behaviours, but many of which are then relegated to the glossing term 'petting' and thereby treated as different from 'real' sex. Here, of course, Schofield adopts a commonsensical viewpoint, although his purpose was neither to analyse commonsensical constructions of what 'sex' is, nor to discuss the different constructions of it held by men and women that Slater and Woodside's research hints at and on which Geoffrey Gorer's work centres. For Gorer, the existence of a 'sexual double standard' constitutes the major way of understanding sexual behaviour, with women seen as having different understandings and different behavioural practices from men. There are similarities here with Chesser's research, which at a number of points implies both that women's orgasmic functioning and sexual desire is different from men's, and also that it thereby constitutes a 'difficulty' that needs to be 'overcome'. The National Survey certainly asked people about a wide variety of behaviours, the vaginal, oral and anal and 'other genital forms of sex', but it still fails to enquire in detail about people's sexual behaviour. For instance, it contains no information on how such genital sexual behaviour interlinks with other erotic and sexual but non-genital behaviour, nor does it investigate whether and in what ways these 'patterns' might differ with a change of partners, or on different occasions. Even at the level of describing the behavioural this research is highly limited, while, as I have already noted, it excludes meaning altogether and eschews analysis except at the most basic of levels.

Behind this general shared taken-for-grantedness about what 'sex' is and how its constituent behaviours articulate, lies the even more fundamental assumption of heterosexuality as axiomatically 'the norm', as 'what is natural' in sexual terms because seen as entirely innate. In Slater and Woodside's and Chesser's research there is no mention of any homosexual behaviour or partners at all, and while Schofield notes that a significant proportion of both boys and girls knew others involved in homosexual sexual experiences, with a smaller group being so involved themselves, this is not explored in his research, which focuses instead on 'sex' – that is, heterosex. Gorer's *Exploring English Character* notes that most of those people who were 'not interested in sex' were actually homosexually involved (and thus were 'interested in sex', although not of a heterosexual kind), although the later *Sex and Marriage* completely ignores the existence of homosexual behaviour and the overlapping of homosexual and heterosexual experiences and feelings in a large number of people's lives. Only the National Survey does not proceed from the assumption that the 'sex' that is being inquired about is necessarily heterosexual. However, it too ends by relegating everything else to an implicit 'and also' status through its concern with fixing people to 'lifestyles'that are conceived as heterosexual or, for a tiny minority, gay male, with lesbian 'lifestyles' being too numerically insignificant even to be discussed.[3]

The taken-for-grantedness of (heterosexual) sex links to a further related assumption, that of the synonymity of heterosexuality and specifically penetrational forms of sex. Thus Slater and Woodside are concerned almost exclusively with 'intercourse', looking at modes of its 'performance' on a weekly basis and people's assumption of a norm in its performance and their own claimed adherence to such a norm. Similarly, Chesser discusses mainly intercourse within marriage; and although women's perception of the absence or insufficiency of 'petting' behaviours – that is, non-penetrational forms of love-making – provides one of the key reasons they give for sexual dissatisfaction, this is ignored by him. In some contrast and perhaps because he was concerned particularly with teenagers, Schofield does note the different behaviours and stages of 'petting' activities, but then still conceptualizes these as falling short of 'sex', that is, penetration. Gorer construes the point at which people first 'had sex' as synonymous with first having intercourse, while his discussion of 'rates in intercourse' is precisely that, not rates of sexual behaviour as such but instead rates of penetration.[4] Again, the National Survey asks about a wider range of activities – vaginal, oral and anal sex and other genital contact – although as noted above it still remains concerned with what is 'high risk', the specifically genital rather than 'sexual experience' or 'sexual contact' defined more widely.

These ideas and assumptions collectively add up to variations on a 'drive reduction' approach,[5] one in which 'sex' (that is, that unspecified behaviour that is actually implicitly heterosexual and penetrational) constitutes a basic need or drive that requires a regular outlet of the right kind. Slater and Woodside, for example, postulate sexual attraction in terms of a kind of low-key fetishism and associate it with repressed emotions within the unconscious, while Chesser proposes that women's lack of orgasm and the refusal of sex leads to emotional and other stresses. Schofield's research is concerned with people younger than the age at which long-term partnerships have been formed, and is more concerned with the deleterious effects of regular sexual *activity* than of abstinence, and it also sees teenage sexual activity – the 'early starters' – as somehow odd or deviant. Gorer's work explores evidence for the commonly-held view that neuroticism is the outcome of withdrawal as a form of contraception, but with palpable reluctance has to conclude that correlations of neuroticism against different forms of birth control lend no support for this view. Only the National Survey avoids a 'drive reduction' approach, although this seems due as much to the absence of a discernible interpretational stance as to any principled rejection of such ideas, for its claimed social constructionism is barely noticeable within the text of its books and articles.

Conventional understandings of sexual behaviour within heterosexual relationships are typically predicated upon the assumption of a 'natural' sexual division of labour that assigns different 'roles' in sexual encounters between men and women, a division that can be summarized in stereotypical ideas about male sexual 'activity' and female 'passivity'. Related to this is the accompanying supposition that the different sexual responses of men and women to penetrational sex are the product of constitutional differences.[6] In this regard, Slater and Woodside propose that women are less successful in their adaptation to 'sex' than men, evidenced in their lower rates of orgasm and their generally greater levels of dissatisfaction with sex in marriage; and here Slater and Woodside apparently discern some common unchanging 'it' that both men and women experience (or ought to), which is somehow independent of the particular relationship and the particular ways that each couple do 'it' together. Chesser proposes something very similar, seeing any orgasmic failure in women as the product of changing physiological capacity rather than of the specificities of their experience of love-making or of their partners' sexual in/abilities and concerns. Similarly, Schofield's research notes a number of differences between the sexes: that the sexually active girls most often are so within the context of a sustained relationship, while the sexually active boys are more likely to be involved in a variety of casual relationships; and that more girls than boys do not enjoy their first or even repeated sexual experiences. Gorer's research centres a 'sexual double standard', seeing women as different in sexual behaviour and even more so in attitude from men, and thereby of course treating them as different from an assumed norm that is actually set by *male* behaviour and *male* attitude. Again, the National Survey takes a different approach to sexual divisions of labour, in the sense of asking respondents both 'what they did' and also 'what partners did to them'. But by failing to situate genital and penetrative behaviours in a more general context of sexual conduct, the actually fully reciprocal nature of many heterosexual sexual practices is glossed over by behavioural terms that, by definition, are associated with a division of labour that conventionally assigns 'passivity' to women and 'activity' to men, and this is particularly so regarding penetrational activities.

These different surveys refer to changes in expectations concerning sexual behaviour and sexual pleasure occurring over time. The most obvious example is Chesser's discussion of changes across different age cohorts, although Schofield's research is premised on exploring the apparently different behaviour of young people in the 1960s as compared with earlier generations, while Gorer's work notes the increase in the numbers of women thinking that sex is important when evaluating their marital happiness. However, and with the partial exception of Chesser's work, all of these surveys – including, astonishingly, the National Survey, with its central concern with sexual change, transmission and control – *assume* rather than investigate change over time. The surveys see sexual change starting from relatively repressed and anti-pleasure ideas about sex in a relatively 'safe' context, and moving in the direction of more liberated and pleasure-based views, but in a relatively 'unsafe' context either morally or with regard to health or both. However, in spite of their 'eye on the times' stance, the major change that occurred in sexual attitudes and sexual behaviour over the time-period of these surveys is hardly recognized by them.

This is the change that 'Little Kinsey' and also Mass-Observation's earlier work on the birth-rate had both centred: the changes to women's sexual expectations and women's sexual behaviours. The earlier surveys all contain either ignored or under-theorized findings in this regard, while the National Survey excludes such information altogether. Thus, Slater and Woodside comment on women's unfamiliarity with the word 'orgasm', but do not seriously consider the possibility that beyond the unfamiliarity with the word might be an unfamiliarity with the experience nor relate this to women's lesser satisfaction with their marriages than men. Chesser notes the general problem of researchers using terms and words to investigate sexual behaviour that people may not understand or be alienated by, but does not link this with women's incomprehension or in/experience of orgasm. Schofield's research is aware that more girls than boys express disappointment and lack of pleasure regarding their initial and indeed subsequent sexual encounters, but neither discusses this nor relates it to other research (e.g. by Kinsey or by Masters and Johnson), which had already problematized the penetrational model of heterosexual stereotype. Gorer's work brings together many of these themes, noting women's 'difference' from men in their sexual behaviour and even more their sexual attitudes, their lesser emphasis on the importance of sexual enjoyment, and their considerably lesser experience of orgasm in sexual relationships. However, Gorer assumes a norm constituted by male experiences and practices to which women had not yet attained, and ignores any consideration of the behavioural and interactional dynamics involved, the meanings and feelings that people bring to and invest in the sexual behaviours they do and do not do.

These related ideas and themes provide the implicit theory of the British sex surveys and it almost exactly replicates publicly articulated assumptions and stereotypes. What is surprising is the extent of this overlap between the 'scientific' and the 'commonsense', the almost complete failure in these researches to subject to detailed investigation precisely what 'sex' consists of. It is this failure to research what people were/are doing and not doing and the meanings that this had/have for them that prevents these surveys from coming to grips with social and sexual change. This concern with change and how best, methodologically and substantively, to explore, describe and explain it, is a topic to which I return in Section Three in the context of my discussion of Shere Hite's research. 'Little Kinsey' too fails to problematise 'sex'; nonetheless it does highlight in interesting ways Mass-Observation's more general, and by 1949 long-standing, perception of a change in women's attitudes and behaviours, a change that encompassed the expectations that women had about their lives, their marriages and children, and of the part to be played by sex and sexual pleasure within this. In this sense 'Little Kinsey' centres social change and the part played by women's changing ideas about sex. The full text of 'Little Kinsey' follows in Section Two. Like the other sex surveys discussed here, it provides its readers with a framework of ideas concerning sexual conduct, and, by locating its findings within this framework, it provides an implicit but still highly theorised account of sexual behaviour and attitude. In Section Three I discuss its theorization of the sexual in the context of its distinctive methodological approach, for 'Little Kinsey's' use of 'the survey' form is very different from the sex surveys which followed it. As Section Three argues, the closest comparison is not in fact between 'Little Kinsey' and these mainstream sex surveys, but rather between 'Little Kinsey' and the feminist sex surveys carried out by Shere Hite from the 1970s to the 1990s.

Notes

1 For feminist work offering rather different overviews of a wide range of popular pronouncements, see Lesley Hall (1991) *Hidden Anxieties* and Margaret Jackson (1994) *The Real Facts of Life.*

2 Useful although very different overviews of this wider discourse are to be found in Frank Mort (1987) *Dangerous Sexualities: Medico-Moral Politics in England Since 1830;* and Sheila Jeffreys (1985) *The Spinster and Her Enemies: Feminism and Sexuality 1880–1930,* and (1990) *Anticlimax: A feminist perspective on the sexual revolution.* See also Jeffrey Weeks (1981/1989) *Sex, Politics and Society* and Lesley Hall (1991) *Hidden Anxieties.* The right to name 'what was going on' with regard to sex and sexuality has become hotly contested and highly politicized territory within contemporary academic writing, as witnessed by the enormous interpretational, and sometimes 'factual', differences between these accounts, and particularly between those of Jeffreys and Weeks.

3 In the two books, the text continually slides from ' homosexuality' to 'gay men', with the authors apparently not even noting that they do this.

4 Although it is at least likely that the respondents themselves were replying in terms of a more complex sexual repertoire than the researchers were inquiring about.

5 The classic critique of 'drive reductionist' ways of thinking and presentation of an interactionist alternative is John Gagnon and William Simon's (1973) highly-influential *Sexual Conduct.*

6 As I have noted, it is a version of this that leads the National Survey researchers to define the vagina as women's 'sexual organs'.

'Little Kinsey': Mass-Observation's Sex Survey of 1949

Editorial Annotations

[word/s] indicates either a doubtful reading of the original text, or an editorial insertion using material from elsewhere in the 'Little Kinsey' manuscripts

[....] indicates a gap in the original text or the editorial omission of repititions

Preface

The present report by Mass-Observation, the 18th it has published, breaks rather new ground, not only for Mass-Observation but for social research in this country generally.

A report of this character is liable to lead to considerable controversy. Accuracy of method is particularly difficult. And the prejudices which all factual reports evoke from biased persons are likely to be especially acute in dealing with the present subject.

Although closely associated with Mass-Observation since its inception, I happen to have had no direct part in this survey of sex life in Britain. So, perhaps, a brief word here may clarify certain points both from the position of one with inside knowledge and one without direct interest in the outcome of the particular case.

In the first place, it cannot be too emphatically stated that this is not an attempt to do a British Kinsey Report. The Kinsey investigation lasted for years and covered 12,000 people. It relied on exhaustive methods of interviewing – so exhaustive that it has been severely criticised on the grounds of method. The Kinsey sample has also been severely criticised by Crossley, Gallop and others on the grounds that it is not representative. Nevertheless, Kinsey has lifted the lid off problems which before have seldom or never been discussed from any sort of factual basis.

The present report attempts both something less and something more than Kinsey. The less is evident to the most casual reader. Here he will find none of those gigantic tables of correlations or imposing bibliographies. On the other hand, here he may find more of the actuality, the real life, the personal stuff of the problem, freed from an excess of methodological and statistical background. In subjects of this character, no known method of social research at present produces results which can be called statistically accurate on any far-reaching analysis. On the contrary, in seeking after such a superficial and easily misleading validity of the exact percentage, the human material behind the figures can easily be lost – as it is, I think, in parts of the Kinsey Report.

In the second place, this report requires special comment with regard to its finances and origins. For a very long time Mass-Observation has been wanting to do a survey of this character, just as from the very beginnings of Mass-Observation we have been wanting to study other broad and fundamental problems. It has seldom been possible to do what we want, because money has usually only been forthcoming to make practical or consumer research studies of a short-term nature. Or, during the war, to do ad hoc investigations for the Government. We have always been glad to undertake this work. No social research organisation should ignore the every-day problems of practical life, economics and administration. But far too seldom have we had the opportunity to carry out fundamental research in fields where, for various reasons, the technique which we have developed over the past twelve years would contribute something special. In the present instance, once the Kinsey Report had been published in America the idea of work on this particular subject became suddenly fashionable in England. Even so, it is remarkably difficult to get funds to carry out anything which is realistic and not embedded in academic qualifications. The *Sunday Pictorial*'s offer to buy newspaper rights in the survey, therefore, made our task much easier.

For this, we are deeply grateful to the *Sunday Pictorial*. It left us entirely free to do the survey in any way we liked. In character and presentation it differs in no way from many other[s] of our published reports. The *Sunday Pictorial* had the right to read this report in the first place, and from it to extract material for a series of articles. This they have done. In the past dozen years Mass-Observation has dealt, I think, with practically every national daily, weekly and monthly, as well as with innumerable local and technical papers. One of the greatest difficulties has always been to prevent many of these papers from presenting our material in a manner liable to over-emphasize certain points or distort the over-all emphasis – e.g. by sub-editing our phrases, putting in cross-heads or editorial commentary. The *Sunday Pictorial* played the game by our results, and have (as far as Mass-Observation is concerned) provided an object lesson of editorial good manners.

The scale of this survey is very much less than that of Kinsey. It has been carried out by only two dozen whole-time investigators, talking to 2,052 people, watching [many more], with additional information from about [450] voluntary observers, over a total period of months. It is essentially a preliminary reconnaissance of the field. It makes no claim to be any more than that. For Mass-Observation, the reconnaissance has been invaluable and we now see our way clearly to making much fuller studies with the machinery of investigation already established and the numerous co-operative contacts already made. It remains to be seen if there is anyone ready to finance what is next required – a very extensive survey carrying on from where this one leaves off, yet still realistic and alive and in touch, not pedagogically concerned with fractional differences and decimal distinctions in place of deep meanings and detailed understanding.

The work throughout has been assisted by the helpful advice of several people who have specialised in the study of sex from various points of view. They have assisted in planning the research and have made many helpful comments on the presentation of the material and the conclusions drawn from it. They are not in any way to be held responsible for the report as a whole, but the report has certainly benefited from their generous interest and in nearly every case the suggestions they have made have been adopted. We therefore have gratefully to thank them.

Tom Harrisson, 8 June 1949

Part A, The Survey

Chapter One: Sex Surveyed

The first problem confronting Mass-Observation when it undertook to make a survey of sex was, quite simply, 'is it possible?'. Kinsey in America had already achieved a detailed investigation into the sex habits of the American male. But it seemed likely that English people, less accustomed to questioning, and living in a social atmosphere less heavily charged with the publicity of sex, would prove a more difficult proposition.

It was partly because of these doubts that we decided, reluctantly, more or less to by-pass sex habit for the time being, instead to confine ourselves largely to the study of attitudes. Other equally important reasons for this decision were the limitations of time and money, necessitating concentration on one main aspect of sex, as well as, above all, our conviction that a picture of habit alone, detached from its dynamic context of motive and opinion, is liable to be to some extent misleading. In order not to fall into the opposite trap of producing a sketch of attitudes totally unsupported by the relevant facts of behaviour, we planned to supplement our large-scale survey of attitudes with a smaller investigation into the sex habits of a single group, not necessarily representative of people in general; Mass Observation's National Panel of Voluntary Observers (note 1), a group of people accustomed to regular questioning on all aspects of their life and outlook, proved suitable for this purpose. In addition we intended to carry out a penetrative observational investigation into the social set-up of sex in two study areas – in this report called 'Churchtown' and 'Steeltown' – chatting informally with inhabitants, observing pubs, dance halls, parks etc., interviewing officials, generally penetrating (note 2) deeply, probing into the life of the area.

These were three of the [four] main facets of our scheme: a national sample of attitudes to sex – forming the basic framework to the survey; the sex habits of a single group; and the study of our investigators into varying social patterns of sex. The fourth aspect that we felt necessary to investigate at least superficially was the nature of contemporary opinion forming influences; following up on this we sent postal questionnaires to groups of randomly selected doctors, teachers, and clergymen; we also attempted to collect a sample of the popular literature of sex. Appendix 3 (note 3) discusses in detail the scope and methodology of the whole survey.

Plans for surveys are relatively easy to make; it is more difficult to carry them out, and an even greater problem to decide whether or not they have proved successful. But preliminary piloting of questionnaires soon showed at least that most British people are willing – even pleased – to talk about sex to an unembarrassed interviewer. Throughout our survey we were constantly surprised by the contrast between our own initial expectation of inhibition, embarrassment and rebuff – and the friendly and co-operative manner with which questions were answered. Of all the 2,052 people interviewed, fewer than 20 (less than 1%) refused to continue once the questionnaire's emphasis on sex had been disclosed. On the contrary, 11% agreed to give their name and address in order that they might answer later questions of a more intimate and personal nature. During the whole survey there were no 'scenes' or incidents more unpleasant than that involving the very untypical middle class housewife, who terminated her interview before it had properly begun, by saying that: *"We never mention the word sex in the class of society I belong to."* (68 year old housewife, Oxford).

If willingness to talk freely and co-operatively is a guide to honesty, then for the most part our results genuinely reflect at least what people think they think. Glibness, on the other hand, may conceal a tendency to give the socially correct answer; it may be quicker and less embarrassing, for instance, to say that extra-marital relations are 'disgusting' than to confess to a more unconventional opinion. It is most unlikely that our results are unaffected by this prestige tendency to give the 'correct' reply – particularly since many people are at least partly unaware of their 'dishonesty'. On the other hand, it is often possible to detect distortion at whatever level of conversation it occurs; the M-O technique of broadly framed open-end questions with replies recorded verbatim is partly designed to counter this problem. It is possible to weigh up each reply thoroughly, setting it in its context of the tenor of the whole interview, as well relating it to the general background of the respondent. Assessing and reassessing our material in this way, both investigators and analysts felt that results, on the whole, represented what people think – in so far as they are themselves aware of their own opinions.

On the subject of honesty, the final word had best come from an outside source. One of the expert board of Assessors (note 4) that M-O persuaded to advise it on this survey spent a morning with a regular M-O investigator, not only watching interviews, but also making notes himself. He reported:

> *"It proved possible to question people on their attitudes to sex, & their replies seem, on the whole, to have been fairly honest. But even so, our investigation inevitably has many limitations. It was intended only as a piloting survey and as such the field it covered was deliberately narrowed; but even as a survey of sex attitudes is by no means comprehensive. It is essentially a superficial survey, incapable of pen-*

etrating deeply into the dynamics of sexual attitudes and feelings. In addition we were only able to cover attitudes to the broader aspects of sex, and to its most prominent institutions – marriage, divorce and prostitution. We have only indirect measures, for instance, of [...]opinion on the less socially acceptable sources of sex outlet – notably homosexuality and masturbation. Moreover, carrying out a survey which is unprecedented in this country, our inexperience inevitably led to errors, largely of terminology, which later investigations should be better able to avoid. But above all, future surveys on the subject of sex will be emboldened by the knowledge that it is possible – at least for a stranger who is himself not embarrassed – to question people on almost any aspect of sex. Had we realised this earlier we would have extended our survey to include popular attitudes to homosexuality and masturbation".

But although most people have shown themselves prepared to speak freely about sex, this does not mean that the tradition of British reticence on this subject is a popular figment. Many lengthy interviews retained a faint suggestion of uneasiness lurking behind them, sometimes a barely perceptible suggestion of relief when all the questioning was over; and most started off with something of an initial show of surprise or embarrassment, even when the firmly matter of fact tone of the interview quickly transformed this into interest and even pleasure. Our questions quite clearly elicited interesting reactions not only between types of personalities, but often also within single individuals; many people are anxious and pleased to discuss sex – but remain faintly uneasy in a discussion which they seem otherwise to enjoy. Outside the sphere of the interview, the contrast between the two reactions could be compared with the embarrassed need to turn sex into a joke before it can be discussed – the eagerness with which the jokes are bandied and received.

Later chapters of this report will show how this conflict between co-existent desiring and fearing appears in attitudes to most of the sexual topics covered by our questionnaire. One occasion when this contradiction became particularly apparent was where we tried to assess the extent to which people are prepared to recognise the importance of sex to themselves. The atmosphere of emotionality and interest in which so many of the interviews were conducted suggested that people must attach a high degree of importance to sex; so did the constant insistence that sex is 'natural'. Yet when asked explicitly whether it was possible to be happy 'without some form of sex-life' only 1 in every 3 said that sex was a vital part of a contented life; throughout replies to this and other questions ran what seemed to be a suspicion that sex for its own sake and in its own right and irrespective of the conventional limitations of marriage, frequency or nature, is something to be deprecated as undesirable, perhaps distasteful, often nasty. This distrust of sex, sometimes spoken, sometimes unspoken, seems to lie behind much of the opposition to birth control and sex education, certainly to prostitution and extra-marital relations. It is particularly frequent amongst older people, church-goers, and the less well educated; and its religious derivation seems fairly clear. A phrase particularly common amongst the group of clergymen we questioned was 'self-control'; it is their fear of sex 'uncontrolled', warring uneasily with the recognition of the inevitability and healthiness of sex, that features amongst the most striking results of our survey.

Notes

1. [The] Mass-Observation National Panel is a group of about 1,000 voluntary observers, some of whom have been replying to questions more or less regularly for more than 10 years. Unrepresentative in that they are, as a group, more than usually intelligent and well educated, they are invaluable in their willingness and ability to give an honest and detailed account of their opinions and behaviour. [...] To some extent it was possible to check up on the extent to which they are unrepresentative by relating their attitudes to sex to those of the general population.
[2. The notion of 'functional penetration' became a key Mass-Observation term and was borrowed from research carried out by Oscar Oeser, as discussed in Section One.]
[3. The planned Appendix 3 was unfortunately never written.]
[4. This assessor was Cyril Bibby.]

Part B, The Mechanics of Sex

Chapter Two: The Facts of Life

Present-day opinion tends to spotlight sex education as essential to the normal growth of sex attitudes. Partly for this reason we set out to discover not only what people thought of sex instruction, but also how they themselves had found out about sex. How did the children of the last generation discover the 'facts of life'?

Of the 2,052 people comprising our national street sample, only one in every six (16% of the total) claimed to have received any sex education; in fact precisely 18% had actually received instruction from relatively general sources of mother, father, doctor, father, schoolteacher, or clergyman. Of the remainder, most had 'picked up' their sex knowledge – from other children, from work-mates, off the street corner, just by keeping eyes and ears open. Out of every 100 persons questioned:

25 said, more or less, that they had 'picked up' their sex knowledge
13 had heard from other children
12 said it came 'naturally', or by experience
11 had been instructed by their mother
 8 had found out from reading
 6 had been instructed by their father
 6 "   "   "   "   "   teacher
 6 had learnt from work-mates
 5 had learnt from getting married
 4 "   "   "   the Armed Forces
10 mentioned other sources of knowledge (other relations, fiancées, etc.)
(nb. a few people had gained their knowledge from more than one source).

Nearly a third of those under 25 had received some sort of relatively formal sex education, compared with only a twelfth of the over 45s – so that the practice of imparting sex knowledge would seem to have been on the increase for some decades at least. It seem to be more usual to tell the 'facts of life' to girls than to boys, a result consistent with 1943 Board of Education statistics which showed that about three girls' elementary schools include sex instruction in their syllabus, for every one in boys' schools (note 1). Above all, education is most common amongst the group that has had a full time education up to the age of 17 or more (which of course includes a high proportion of young people) although even in this group casual methods of discovering sex are slightly more frequent than the more formal sources of father, mother and schoolteacher. The schoolyard is more often the source of sex instruction than the class-room, the street corner more often than the home. The biology class atmosphere is strikingly absent from these replies:

> *"Oh, I heard it knocking about with the boys"* (47 year old building labourer, Newport)

> *"I picked it up on the street corner with my mates"* (38 year old unemployed porter, Exeter)

> *"Just picked it up, you know. In the gutter, more or less"* (26 year old unemployed street metal maker, Wembley)

> *"When you're kids you prick up your ears and listen-in to your mothers talking"* (47 year old joiner's wife, York)

Usually there is a matter-of-fact ring of acceptance about this sort of admission, that is the way sex knowledge used to be acquired, and more could not have been expected of the parents of the last generation. But sometimes a more wistful or resentful note creeps in: -

> *"I just picked it up from friends. I don't say it's the best way, mind you. But you can't expect your mother or father to sit down and tell you such things."* (18 year old Building Labourer, Worcester)

> *"I learnt in a very horrible and rotten manner"* (35 year old woman, factory worker, Hendon)

On the whole it is only the more elderly, forgetful perhaps of their earlier difficulties, who are completely satisfied with the more casual methods of self-instruction. An Old Age Pensioner, for instance, remarks complacently:

> *"I had no sex education. I allowed nature to take its course, and it never let me down."* (68 year old Old Age Pensioner, Peterborough)

Precisely what is meant by the 'natural' method is obscure, sometimes it seems to be the way of experience, sometimes of observation – but more often it probably just implies the realisation of blurred memories, conferring respectability on more devious and disreputable sources; older people are particularly inclined to mention 'natural' sources:

> *"Well it just come to me, natural, mixing with other girls."* (48 year old engineer's wife)

> *"I picked it up natural. We were farmers you see. And then a lad that read the Bible would find out that way. There are a lot of things in the Bible to learn from."* (60 year old working man, retired, Doncaster)

> *"I joined the Territorial Army, and I went to my first camp at 17, and a young girl in Swansea took me down a back alley, and she made all the advances; that's how I learnt"* (27 year old baker, Peterborough)

> *"Nobody taught me, they didn't need to. I had eyes in my head. Mind you, I've always lived on a farm – I don't know how townspeople would go on."* (52 year old farmer, Tadcaster)

This sort of casual gleaning of sex information is more or less typical. It is clear that most people – of the present adult generation, at least – have been left to stumble for themselves upon the 'facts of life'. For those to whom not only formal instruction but 'street corner' sources were denied, it was literally a matter of putting two and two together on the basis of whatever information they could discover. One in twelve said, for instance, that he had got his facts from reading; literature provides an extensive and varied source of information for those who set out in earnest after knowledge:

> *"I learnt from such books as Havelock Ellis – which was in the house. I knew about sex when I was eight."* (30 year old ex-naval officer, private income, Oxford)

> *"By the daily paper"* (49 year old hospital porter, Denbigh)

> *"I got hold of a little book called the 'Red Light' and it puts it all in John Blunt language"* (26 year old salesman, Redhill)

Just over half of Mass-Observation's National Panel mention books as one source of their sex knowledge. Medical books – found either at home or in libraries – are the usual literary source in this more than usually well-educated group, and closely followed by biology and physiology textbooks.

Most frequent authors mentioned by name are Havelock Ellis and Marie Stopes. The following is a list of all books and specific types of books specified. Those starred occur more than once or twice:

*Havelock Ellis
Norman Haire
Van de Velde
*Dictionaries
*Encyclopaedia

*Books on Sex Hygiene, Sex Instruction Manuals
Aristotle
*Marie Stopes
W. Bowen-Partington (writing in 'Health and Strength')
Red Light
'Health Manuals'
"The Household Family Doctor's Book"
*Physiological Books, Natural History Books, Biology Books
*Freud
*Kenneth Walker
Illustrated Medical Dictionary
L. N. Fowler
*Bible
'The Home Doctor'
Max Hodam
Shakespeare
'Grown up novels'
A. S. Neill
Kraft Ebing
Magnus Hirshfield
Dr. Gray 'Men, Women and God'
Huxley
Bertrand Russell

It is in their tendency to refer to books for information on sex that this middle-class National Panel group seems most to differ from the street sample. But this difference is to some extent more apparent than real. The Panel group is above average in its level of education and more able to search out knowledge from books – but on the whole their sex reading only supplements other less respectable methods of digging out information. Most of this group – but very few of the street sample – mention two ways in which they found out about sex, and the non-reading methods are similar to those mentioned by the street sample: casual picking up of sex facts from other children and haphazard sources is the most frequent method, and only one in three has had any sort of relatively formal instruction. Here, for instance, is an account given by a woman to whom reading was just one of several ways in which she discovered the 'facts of life':

> *"I remember asking my mother where babies came from when I was about 8 years old. With my brothers and sisters I was in bed with measles. She said 'Ask the doctor' which I did, whereupon he merely laughed and said something about 'When you're older'.*
>
> *When about 12 or 13 I was on top of a bus with my mother when I asked why only married women had children. Some unsatisfactory reply caused me to say I would have a child if I wished, married or*

no. I remember the incident because of my mother's unaccountably angry condemnation of me.

I hunted among my father's large library for information and found a book on the 'Care of Babies'. I read it in bed and hid it under the mattress where mother found it and taxed me. I knew not what to say and shrank with embarrassment and a sense of guilt.

At fourteen a school friend told me her sister was going to have a baby. We discussed the subject and she said she was sure it was in her tummy. We assumed it would come out of the navel, that that was the purpose of the navel.

I became an apprentice at B.... (a large London store) and 'lived in', sharing a room with three other girls. One of these decided to become a nurse. One summer evening on returning to this room when work was done I found Phyllis (the would-be nurse) lying on her bed with the other two girls seated each side of her. They were studying a catalogue from which Phyllis was to choose her uniform and accessories.

They commenced to giggle and I flew over to share the fun. Phyllis pointed to an illustration of a pessary (a rubber sheet, 'French letter') amid more giggles. My bewilderment was obvious and with much guffawing they told me its purpose.

I was stunned. For many days afterwards I went about my work in a state of trance, obsessed by this horrifying information. I was nearly seventeen, incredibly foolishly innocent, and had hitherto scorned 'boys'. (Probably late in developing)

I was now horrified at such intimacy with part of the body associated with 'dirt'. On account of this information I took it for granted that a man's penis was normally long and rigid, and I had no knowledge of erection until after marriage at 23.

I think I instinctively connected the correct method of birth with the sex act after learning the above information from Phyllis." (52 year old housewife, member of M-O Panel)

Whether or not her attitude has any connection with the way in which she found out about sex, or with her protracted blindness to sex facts, this woman still retains something of her initial distaste at the 'dirtiness' of sex. Asked whether she though that sex could be in any way harmful, she replied:

"Fragmentary conversations bring to light that sex proves disappointing to the young wife after a time, because husbands merely use them and are not concerned with their partner feeling any satisfaction. With older women it is tolerated as one of life's burdens."

And an elderly male member of Mass-Observation's National Panel describes an unfortunate blending of 'literary and gutter' sources of information:

"I had no sex education, what I learned was picked up from bigger boys in a vulgar way. From them I learned masturbation which nearly ruined me; fortunately, someone knew what I was about and put a leaflet in my way, which I read and took to heart – just in time to prevent me from becoming a waster or imbecile. That was the only bit of advice I ever had." (68 year old retired man, Panel member)

It would be interesting to discover precisely what this leaflet said about masturbation. In the course of our survey we collected information and literature of the type liable to fall into unspecialized hands, and answered advertisements in sex interest weeklies. One of these advertisement replies produced a pamphlet entitled 'Sexual Neurasthenia (Functional Genital Weaknesses) and Mental Inefficiency'. A glance through the pamphlet shows its main interest to be, in more simple words, the sexual ill-effects of masturbation. It introduces discussion with a quotation from Carpenter's *The Intermediate Sex* (note 2):

"To prolong the period of continence in a boy's life is to prolong the period of growth. This is a simple physiological law, and a very obvious one; and, whatever other things may be said in favour of purity, it remains perhaps the most weighty. To introduce sensual and sexual habits – and one of the worst of them is self-abuse – at an early age is to arrest growth, both physical and mental. And what is even more, it means to arrest the capacity for affection. All experience shows that the early outlet towards sex cheapens and weakens affectional capacity."

And the Preface follows up these warnings:

"Thousands of people of all ages have applied to me for relief from the evil consequences of an all too prevalent habit, and so convincingly have these appeals revealed to me the long struggle which has nearly always taken place before the appeal is made, that I have considered the necessity of preparing this little book in the hope that it will bring consolation to thousands of sufferers from the effects of self-abuse showing them that remedy is not only possible, but not difficult, provided the right methods are adopted. I want to convince them that not only can the habit itself be overcome, but that the deleterious results can also be repaired.

"Unfortunately, the habit to which I refer has, on the one hand, been denounced as a heinous sin. This method of censure not only helps to depress the victim already reduced to a state of mental castigation and nervous debility, but it makes him reluctant to apply for help, because of the shame which, he has been told, attached to his weakness"

In spite of the disclaiming of the 'sinfulness' of masturbation, the whole tone of the pamphlet underlines the physical ill-effects of the habit. Here, for instance, is a letter included as testimonial from a youth who has now been 'cured of sexual weakness':

"Some time ago I received particulars of your course of Physical Culture.

I am in my twentieth year, and wish to come under your care for the correction of a very pernicious habit.

I first became addicted, in ignorance, to the habit of self-abuse at the age of about 13 years. Between the ages of 15 and 17, it became an almost daily habit, and even now, when I have begun to realise what I am doing, I fall twice and sometimes three times a week, in spite of my efforts to check it.

The result is that I am now well on the way to becoming a nervous wreck.

I have been puzzled, and not a little perturbed, to observe that whereas in my schooldays I was keen-witted and clever, I am now becoming quite a duffer.

Other effects of the habit are lack of concentration, lack of self-confidence, weak will-power, 'nervousness', self-consciousness, and shyness, the 'inferiority complex', general mental laziness. I am also given to worrying over trifles, and suffer occasionally from constipation and neuralgia.

My eyes too seem weak, they 'water' freely in the cold weather and even in a light wind, and in moments of embarrassment.

Any other particulars you may require I shall be pleased to give, as I am confident that you will do all in your power to put me on the clean and decent path once more.

P.S. I have given you my weight and measurements in the space provided on the consultation form, as I wish to have your opinion of these. I have an idea that I am rather under-developed for my age. Is this so?

"Last letter:-
"I have now completed your course, and beg to render my sincerest thanks for the great improvement which has taken place in my condition.

I consider the day that I decided to take up your course as the turning point of my life, and I look forward to the future with joyous anticipation.

Three months ago I was practically a nervous wreck; nervous, self-conscious, and lacking grit and will-power, and all those qualities which mark the difference between the man and the imbecile.

Today I find myself a well-set up youngster, with an erect carriage and a firm step, bright-eyed, and fresh complexioned – a picture of health and energy.

I had never done anything in the way of physical exercises before I took up your course, but I found your exercises both pleasant and interesting.

I shall be grateful, now that I have completed the course, for any hints that you can give me as to how to keep fit, and maintain the improvement I have derived from the course.

  Believe me,
    Sincerely grateful"

Kinsey found much the same situation in America. In his 'Sexual Behaviour in the Human Male', he writes:

"[...] there are definite taboos against masturbation. These may be fortified with the explanation that masturbation will drive one crazy, give one pimples, make one weak or do some other sort of physical harm. More often masturbation is simply rejected because it is considered un-natural...."

Earlier in his report Kinsey suggests that his material shows no physically harmful outcome of masturbation at however early an age it is begun, and however frequently it is indulged in. Most present day psychiatrists would support his conclusions. Unless ill-effects are a result of information and attitudes of the kind disseminated in the pamphlet quoted above, there would seem to be little rational basis for masturbation anxiety. In any case, whatever its scientific validity, pamphlets of this kind discussing so graphically what is in this case described as the 'evil results of sexual excesses whether solitary, normal or abnormal' (but concentrating particularly on masturbatory 'excess') are likely to be, at the very least, a disturbing document to fall into the hands of an adolescent seeker after sex knowledge.

It is clear that reading matter may not always be a satisfactory way of learning about sex. Even formal instruction – where it is given – is often inadequate or just too late, although the inadequacy is usually accepted in good grace and with sympathy for parents doing what is felt to be an awkward and embarrassing job:

"My mother told me a bit – but it had to be dragged out of her. She once told me nothing was so difficult as having to tell your daughter the facts of life. I learnt a lot more by the back stairs so to speak" (52 year old woman, pig-breeder, Tadcaster)

"My mother told me, but only after my periods had started and I nearly died of fright" (48 year old decorator's wife, Oxford)

> *"I learned from the girls at school. I was always terrified of sex. My mother was always trying to tell me but never quite did".* (47 year old middle-aged woman, private means, Oxford)

Insofar as formal instruction goes, the most usual source of knowledge is the mother of the family – mentioned by one man in fourteen and one woman in seven. Only after her comes the father, and schoolteacher; fathers are most inclined to teach their sons about sex, mothers their daughters. Age differences suggest that the schoolteacher as a source of sex information has been gaining in importance, whilst the mother's position altered less rapidly; mothers are mentioned twice as often in the younger than the older groups, whilst teachers are mentioned 15 times more often. Fathers, meanwhile, have been creeping up at an [increasing] rate. Other relatively formal sources of sex knowledge that are mentioned occasionally are clergymen, employers and doctors. Here, for instance, is a man who went to the parson for information:

> *"When I was 20 I didn't know a thing, and I went to see our parson, and he told me. He put it to me in a nice way, he said 'Do you grow marrows, George?'. I said I did and he told me 'Well, you've got to pollenize marrows to make them grow, haven't you?' and he showed me how it was done. If it is done in a nice way like that I suppose it is all right."* (60 year old shopkeeper, Peterborough)

Like this man, many of those who received some kind of semi-formal instruction had to ask for it first. And – again, like him – some claim that they did not realise until a later date that there was anything to be told. One midwife who was interviewed said that not until her first midwifery case did she realise that men had anything to do with producing babies:

> *"At 26 years of age, I was as ignorant as it was possible to be. The funny part is that I can't imagine how I lived to that age without realising. I wasn't helped in the slightest bit. It makes me howl when I think of it. Even when I started my midwifery training I never thought fathers had anything to do with it, I nearly made an awful blunder asking a woman if her husband had anything to do with it."* (61 year old woman, retired nurse)

And a similar case, this time at second hand:

> *"I think sex education is very wise. It does lessen the ignorance and misery. Why, only the other day a girl I know came to me in a very tearful state, She is 25 and expecting her first baby, and she hadn't the faintest idea what was going to happen – whether it was going to come out under her arms or what. So I told her 'It comes out at the same place as it goes in my dear'. But isn't it awful that any one should be brought up in such ignorance."* (55 year old widow, (532))

These are not extreme cases, but rather milder instances of prolonged ignorance, and do not appear to be by any means rare. Although discovery of sex
facts by 'getting married' seems – from the relative elderliness of the majority mentioning it – to be a dying phenomena, it is still mentioned by one in
every twenty, usually the less 'well-educated' and generally women. A working class housewife, for instance, said:

> *"I didn't know until I was married – all my mother said was 'Behave
> yourself' – and none of the details"* (39 year old grinder's wife, (531))

How far does a later and sudden discovery of sex involve people in unnecessary emotional difficulties, and upset their sexual adjustments? One case,
where this had possibly happened, has already been quoted. Other people –
particularly women – occasionally discuss the shock and fears that they
remember resulting from their belated or haphazard discovery of sex; but this
is not something that is likely to be recalled, or easily spoken of:

> *"I learnt just by myself. I didn't know anything until I started asking
> about it. I lost my parents when I was young, and my grandparents
> never told me anything. I know when I first had my periods I was
> scared to death because I thought you only had that if you had been
> doing anything wrong."* (45 year old engineer's wife, Exeter)

Such spontaneous instances of upsets resulting from sudden haphazard discovery of sex are not frequent and such as they are come almost exclusively
from women – again probably because of the shock of menstruation. Men
appear to have encountered less anxiety, and seem less resentful of their lack
of instruction, perhaps anyway street-corner bandying of sex facts is more
common amongst boys than amongst girls:

> *"I learnt a lot of terrifying things in the factory where I worked, and
> then I learnt afterwards they was all lies. Awful things, the girls used
> to tell me."* (21 year old cycle-viewer's wife, (621))

> *"It just came like a bolt from the blue. It's rather a jar when it comes
> like that and when you're a little sensitive."* (36 year old busker (532))

It seems likely that in some cases an unguarded stumbling upon haphazard
sex facts has had a harmful effect on later development. But feelings on sexual topics are quite clearly much too complex, both in themselves and in their
motivation, to be directly related to other single factors. It is probably too
much to expect that a direct relation between sources of sex knowledge on
the one hand, and attitudes on sexual topics on the other, should emerge statistically. In fact, our correlations do not indicate any statistical relation
between the way people find out about sex, and, for instance, their inclination

to feel that sex is unpleasant or their feelings about extra-marital sex relations; if such a relation does exist it is obscured by other factors. But although statistical evidence is lacking, it is by no means difficult to find individual cases where sex instruction, or the lack of it, seems to have some influence on attitudes. Here, for instance, is a middle-aged twice-married housewife, who received none:

> *"I didn't know the difference between man and woman when I went on my honeymoon. Mother said 'Don't cry, it happens to all women' – that's bad. My first marriage was no good; my second is wonderful."*

A middle aged woman, unmarried and keeping home for her father, vaguely dislikes the idea of marriage:

> *"Marriage always puzzled me, and I had a [feeling] of evasion to the though of it, and also I should hate to have the feeling I was tied to somebody. I think a woman can carve a career out for herself, independent of a man. That's what gets me, people breaking their necks to marry; it doesn't answer sometimes, and then they wish they were single again."*

This woman has stray recollections of the shock that discovering sex meant to her:

> *"I found out when I left school. Things that children say to one another – 'a lady and a gentleman..' – you know how they put it, so crudely. It was such a shock to me. I don't think I ever got over it, because I thought my mother and father would never do such a thing as that."*
> (51 year old housewife, keeps home for Old Age Pensioner, father)

And a housewife and charwoman, coming unexpectedly upon sex information:

> *"I found out from my older sister. I was there when she had her first baby, and I helped her all I could; and then she told me all about how it came to be there. It was an awful shock to me."*

Whether or not as a result of this shock, this woman's attitude to sex is by no means normal either in the emotionality of her attitudes or in her efforts to condone sexuality:

> "(Marriage?) *It's what you make of it, I have been very, very, happy.*
>
> (Birth Control?) *I don't think a child should be stopped from coming, it is conceived by the Holy Ghost and it only comes because God*

grants it ...
(Extra-marital relations?) *Oh, it's disgusting.*

(Impossible to be happy without sex?) *I don't believe in it at all – it's wrong, it's horrible, unless it comes in normal married life, when God says it has to be in order to have children.*

(Is sex wrong?) *It can be. It is, because God says it has to be, and we couldn't have children without – but otherwise it is very wrong and disgusting.*

(Can sex be unpleasant?) *You have to love a man very much in order to enjoy it, it would be impossible to be pleasant with just any man."*

Cases of this kind in our material do not occur frequently, but they are by no means rare, amongst women at least. Interesting as they are as brief case-histories, however, they cannot demonstrate any relation between manner of acquiring sex knowledge, and later adjustment to sex. Even if such a relation should be shown to exist, it might well be a matter not of one thing causing another, but of two things both caused by a third factor – in this case possibly an even earlier reluctance to accept the facts of sex – a capacity for being sexually shocked. Even so, it is interesting that it is much more difficult to discover cases of apparently good sexual adjustment following on after a shocked reception of the 'facts of life'. It seems at least clear that the way sex information is received is important to later adjustment, even if the way that it is imparted remains more doubtfully influential.

Notes

1 See Educational Pamphlet no.119, published in 1943 by the Board of Education
[2 Edward Carpenter's *The Intermediate Sex* was published in 1908 (Allen & Unwin, London); the title essay had been removed, at his publisher's insistence, from his *Love's Coming Of Age*, published in 1896 (Allen & Unwin, London) just after the Oscar Wilde trial. In its day, *The Intermediate Sex* was a radical book that encouraged pride and a determination to live more openly to very many gay men and lesbian women and is an important landmark in the establishment of an open gay presence in Britain.]

Chapter Three: Sex Education

Most people have received no formal sex instruction of any kind, and generally they seem to accept their background with equanimity. But how do they feel about the idea of sex education for the next generation? On most of the topics concerned with sex and sexual morality it is dangerous to generalise about changes in opinion, because of the lack of earlier comparative opinion surveys; on the subject of sex education, however, a change seems fairly clear. During the last few years, official statements on this issue have achieved a somersault, turning the pronouncements of the twenties topsy turvey – and it seems likely that public opinion has followed a similar course.

It is interesting to trace this change of official heart back to its beginnings. In 1914 the [London County Council] passed a resolution banning sex education from their schools – a ban which was lifted a few months ago. Earlier, apparently moved by the same forces as drove the L.C.C. to a new decision, the Ministry of Education had given official sanction to sex education for the young, again reversing an earlier Act. The post-war period has also seen the National Union of Teachers, the Roman Catholic Archbishops, as well as Bishops in England and Wales, all give their blessing to an idea which 20 or 30 years ago was more or less out of the question. Testing official views with a postal questionnaire sent to doctors, teachers and clergymen, our own survey showed that each of these groups are now over-whelmingly in favour of sex education; against the idea were only:

> 1% of the teachers   }
> 5% of the doctors   }   against sex education
> and 10% of the clergymen }

Similarly, only 2% of Mass-Observation's National Panel, more or less representative of middle-class 'progressive' opinion, were opposed to sex education – although an additional 7% had mixed or uncertain views. Sex education is now, officially and professionally at least, respectable.

Whether or not his opinions have followed the same evolutionary course, or been moved by the same forces as those affecting officialdom, 'the man in the street' now finds himself in much the same position as the expert. Three quarters of the general population, represented by our national street sample, are in favour of sex education. Out of say, 100 questioned:

76 were in favour
15 were against
9   had mixed feelings, and had not made up their minds.

Moreover, approval of sex education is as wholehearted as it is widespread. Perhaps one indication that the battle has been won lies in the fact that so very many of the exponents of sex education felt it unnecessary to give reasons for their support. Most content themselves with: *"That's a very good thing", "That's necessary", "I'm all for that"* – a very different form of reply from the more lengthy and elaborated views of the opposite camp. Today it is the opponents of sex education who are on the defensive.

That opposition to sex education may represent a dying outlook is also suggested by its prevalence amongst the old rather than the young; one person in four over the age of 45 is against it – but only one in fourteen of the younger group. Young people, men, the more adequately educated, and non-churchgoers, are most frequently in favour (at all events amongst those groups that we were able to investigate); this is probably because women are usually more inclined than men to cling to old ideas; and throughout our sex survey, we found that non-church-goers were consistently the more in favour of sexual freedom. Lastly, and perhaps most significantly of all, those who themselves received formal sex education were overwhelmingly in favour of it, although a very few had been set against sex education by their own experience of its consequences:-

> *"No, I like it to be taboo. I was brought up in that free way – I went to an experimental school – and I don't approve of it. We had no taboos at all, neither at home nor at school, and I really don't think it's wise. I'm sending my children to a very conventional school now."*
> (38 year old housewife, husband 'in shipping', Reigate)

Personal experience of sex education usually inclines people to favour it, and – equally – experience of 'gutter' sources of sex knowledge is often a reason for advocating more reputable methods of instruction for others. Most people agree with sex education quite simply because they feel that it is often a necessary means of helping the next generation to avoid their own difficulties:-

> *"Everyone should be sex educated. I was brought up in ignorance – I didn't make a fatal mistake, but I might have done."* (30 year old electrician, Hendon)

Although opposition to sex education is stronger in some groups than in others, in all the groups that we were able to isolate it remains very much a minority view. But what the opposition lacks in numbers is easily made up in strength of feeling; there can be little comparison between the relatively complacent acceptance of the favourable majority and the bitter feelings of their opponents. Reasons for objecting to sex education fall into three main groups:

> that it is unnecessary
> that it is distasteful, perhaps immoral
> that it will corrupt the child

In the first and most common of these arguments there is more than a hint of the dragweight of conservatism; there are ways and means of discovering sex without the bother of formal instruction, and in any case what has been good enough for the parents should still suffice for the child:-

> "*I don't agree with it. It can come natural without them being stuffed up with it. I didn't have any, and it came natural to me when I was married.*" (47 year old wife of painter's labourer, Wigan)

And a miner, who said that he had found out himself by going with women, dismissed sex education as :

> "*... a lot of nonsense. They have to find out for themselves.*" (48 year old miner, Wigan)

This miner's use of the imperative 'have', and the feeling that acquiring knowledge about sex is a natural process that is best left undisturbed, both suggest that resistance to sex education is to some extent reinforced by moral strictures. There is even more of this moral tone in the views of those who condemn sex education as not 'nice', even as somehow nasty or disgusting and to that extent wrong:

> "*I don't think it's right myself. We never had it, and I don't think it's nice for kiddies to know about such things.*" (25 year old wife of trimmer in pressed steel works, Oxford)

> "*I don't hold with it. It's disgusting.*" (Old age pensioner's wife, St. Albans)

> "*I don't think they should – they make fun of it. My two boys came home from school laughing and joking about it*" (28 year old bus conductor's wife, Shrewsbury)

Inevitably, moral censure of sex education finally spreads to those who give information, even to the children themselves receiving it:

"I remember my next-door neighbour was going to have a baby and I was talking to her. I'd notice [d] her little girl standing at the front door looking at the sky for some weeks past and I asked her [what] she was looking for. The woman said with a laugh 'Oh, she's been there for weeks looking for the stork bringing the baby'. She obviously thought it very funny, but I was shocked, and said it was being cruel to the child, and that I'd told my children all about babies, and thought it was the kindest and safest thing to do. Well – my little girl used to play with the child next door and about a week later, I heard that this woman had said that her daughter wasn't to play or talk with ours because ours was being brought up to have a vulgar mind."
(Railway driver's wife, aged 48, Worcester)

The third main argument against sex education is that it will corrupt the child. How far this is a conclusion reached through observation and rational deduction, how far it is merely the inevitable end of a train of thought and feeling that began by suspecting sex education of immorality in itself, it is difficult to judge:

"I don't think I agree with it. The children are wicked enough these days ... I've seen things." (49 year old woman, keeps house for her unemployed mother, Manchester)

Sometimes there is an indisputable suggestion of faulty logic:

"Well I don't know what to think. I read a case in the paper yesterday of a girl having a baby at 14, and she had had sex education." (48 year old engineer's wife, Hendon)

But attitudes are meaningful only against a full background of the subject to which they refer. What do people mean by sex education? The battle for instruction may have been won, but the victors are left with the doubtful triumph of ambiguity and internal conflict; how and by whom should the 'facts of life' be given? And what sort of facts?

For most people sex education seems to mean instruction given possibly in the home, but more likely at school. Although only 4% of those who had actually been told about sex by their mother or father denied having received sex education, there remains a certain amount of confusion on this score; for some people sex education can only mean school education and they judge the former according to their views on the latter. In particular this is one source of opposition to sex education, coming from people who feel that parents are the proper people to tell children about sex. For most people, however, puberty is the time for sex instruction, and for this reason it is more or less inevitable that the school should be regarded as a suitable background for it. As many as two-thirds of our street sample suggested 10 or over (usually 13 or 14) as the best years for telling children about sex. As one Exeter man said:

> *"They should be told as they start to change their young natures".* (67 year old Insurance Agent, Exeter)

There is a very prevalent fear of starting sex education too early; 'not too young' is a constantly recurring proviso:

> *"I wouldn't like to tell my child, – but I'd like her to know at school – but not too young"* (27 year old painter and decorator (111))

> *"Every child should know it before leaving school. At about 14."* (58 year old bookstall manager (113))

A fair-sized minority would even postpone sex education till after leaving school:

> *"School-children are too young to go in for that sort of thing."* (75 year old Old Age Pensioner (331))

Of every 100 in our street sample:

14 think sex education should be given as early as possible, or under 6 years.
13 think it should be given up to 10 years
25 "   "   "   "   "   at 11 or 12
29 "   "   "   "   "   at 13 or 14
13 "   "   "   "   "   at 15 or over
6   give mixed or uncertain replies

Women are inclined to suggest an earlier age for sex education than men, probably because they often have menstruation in mind – the need for warning girls of its approach, as well as for informing them of its meaning. And differences between income groups and between the more and the less educated groups in this respect show very clearly the way the wind is blowing; suggesting that sex education should take place before 10 were:

45% of those leaving school after $16\frac{1}{2}$
32% of those leaving school after 15 up to $16\frac{1}{2}$
24% of those leaving school up to 15

Quite clearly, the more education people have themselves, the more they are inclined to accept the idea of sex instruction at a relatively early age. Income differences reflect this educational trend, which emerges once again when street sample views on sex education are compared with those of members of Mass-Observation's National Panel. Of this middle-class group, more than half suggest that the best age of sex education is 'as early as possible', before the age of 6, or as the child asks its questions – almost always implying that such instruction is a matter for the parents: only one in five prefers the school-sounding years of 10 onwards. Of the doctors, teachers and clergymen sent our postal questionnaire, although these were not specifically questioned on the most suitable age for instruction, about a quarter spontaneously insisted that sex education should be carried out in the home, hardly any made the [...] stipulation that this task should be reserved for the school teacher.

Whereas the majority of people still see the issue of sex education in black and white, as a matter simply of for or against, [the] middle classes and the 'expert' accept the basic principle but refine and complicate it with semi-psychological subtleties – it is good for children to be taught about sex, but information should be given in the home, since there it can be both given and received in a more natural manner. Moreover, it is felt that if sex facts are given as simple answers to spontaneous questions, this will avoid the dramatic emphasis that may be inevitable if sex is spot-lighted by specially arranged lessons at school. It is largely on these grounds that the higher educational groups suggest that the home, not the school, is the proper setting for sex education. A 35 year old laboratory technician (Panel member) wrote:

> *"Sex education should bear a small but natural part in the awakening of understanding in the growing child. I deprecate any special emphasis on the subject. It should be started before school age, in answer to the child's questions."*

A 30 year old sales representative:

> *"You can't just start it at some particular age, as you do with algebra. Children should have some sex knowledge before formal education begins."*

And an agricultural specialist:

> *"there should be no need for putting it into a separate category. It should be given as soon as interest is displayed – no fairy tales or gooseberry bushes, please."*

Only a relatively small minority of the general sample have absorbed this idea that parents may be best able to impart sex facts in a natural and unemphatic manner. Amongst this generally less educated group any insistence on parents as the most suitable sex instructors is usually likely to spring from a moral origin – sex education is the parent's duty:

> *"I don't agree with it in school. If a mother won't teach her own daughter it is a poor look-out, I say."* (26 year old railway fireman, Doncaster)

And a clergyman shows a similar tendency to prefer parent-instructors for moral reasons:

> *"I would advocate sex education by the right kind of people. It is the duty of parents to give it."* (64 year old clergyman, York).

But on the whole it is largely from the point of view of social and psychological expediency that sex education is approved and the manner giving it discussed. Morality creeps in chiefly amongst the views of those who disapprove instruction – and also when people are discussing what sort of facts children should be told. Clergymen particularly – as might be expected – are inclined to feel that sex facts should be taught in the framework of morality and religious principles:

> *"Sex education is all right so long as the teacher has a firm grasp of sexual morality, and realises that he is teaching human persons an intensely personal subject, and therefore should guide them into self-discipline as well teach his subject."* (29 year old curate, unmarried)

> *"Sex education is important. But let it be given in the light of God, and not just as biology. Sex is a gift from God."* (43 year old clergyman, unmarried)

To most doctors and teachers, as well as to members of Mass-Observation's National Panel and the majority of the street sample, however, sex education is merely a way of imparting sex knowledge in an entirely factual manner. Sex is just another subject that has to be learnt about, like botany or physics:

> *"Introduce it more or less into the framework of education, not necessarily as sex – more or less as a natural science."* (30 year old Accountant (532))

And for the majority of people who approve [of] sex education, its only relation to morality is that – in the minds of some – it may help to avoid an unwitting display of immorality. Sex knowledge may eliminate a 'mistake':

> *"I'm all for it. It stops a lot of gossip such as 'Mum – where do babies come from?' A child has got to find out some time. And the more they know the more chance there is of going straight."* (23 year old telephonist (531))

Perhaps it is this very factual conception of sex education that gives the 'man in the street', in his role of father, a merited interest in shifting the responsibility for instruction on the teacher. Almost none of the teachers who replied to our questionnaire complained of the difficulties of sex education; parents, on the other hand, are subject to embarrassment and confusions and are probably also more inclined to shift the more difficult aspects of the subject:

> *"It is a very interesting question. My children are all very different. I*

more or less taught them the first facts with the poultry. Those hens! They stand you in good stead. But I have to be very careful with my third child. She thinks things out. Her questions are going to be, how did the egg get into the hen? Everything went all right until I got the cock-bird. Then they say, 'What's he doing, the nasty thing – fighting?' and try to push him off." (45 year old joiner's wife, York)

One mother lays up future difficulties for herself with half-truths:

"I told my little boy that a soul of a baby is planted in Mummy's body by God, and that Mummy has to be ill before she has it. Of course I haven't told him how the soul gets there, but I shall when he is older ..." (40 year old charwoman)

A father procrastinates:

"Some say the parent should teach the children. I had two sons and I must say I found it very difficult. I kept putting it off, then blurted out something." (68 year old retired farmer, Panel member)

And a housewife, frightened and confused when a knowledgeable child comes into contact with her own uninstructed children, would be glad to ward sex off till an even later age:

"I don't like the idea of it all in school. I think they learn that time enough. Now a little boy over that way, he's about 6, and his mummy had gone away to have a baby. He comes over to see me and I said 'Well Jimmy, has Mummy gone away for a holiday' and he said 'Holiday be damned, she's gone to have a baby'. Well there were mine around the table, I didn't know where to put myself or what to say." (48 year old labourer's wife, (322))

Most parents need to be freer from embarrassment and self-consciousness themselves before the home can become a really suitable and adequate scene of introduction. And it is equally clear that parental instructions constitute a major source of resistance in the grand battle of sex education – a battle joined on the issue of whether or not children from an early age should be allowed to absorb the 'facts of life' in a simple and natural way from their own parents in their own homes – irrespective of whether this knowledge is later supplemented by instruction at school. The last 20 years have seen a revolution in public opinion, transforming itself into widespread acceptance of the necessity for some sort of sex education; will the next two decades see an equally fundamental change – this time affecting the manner in which the education is conceived? Perhaps this elderly middle-class woman, one of our street sample, represents opinion as it will be when the next battle has been won?

"It depends on how it's given. If the teacher has a sympathetic insight into life apart from academic knowledge – I have seen the results and it can be very fine. It unfolds all through life, because when you have a little child out for a walk you teach it about the flowers and you teach it about animals. It unfolds naturally up to the adolescent stage when you teach deeper truths with moral principles ... A little girl I knew flung her arms round her mother's neck, and said, 'Oh Mummy, isn't it beautiful to think I'm a little bit of you.' But she always had a beautiful mind."

Chapter Four: Birth Control

One result of leaving sex education to chance on the street corner is that many people are still either ignorant or inadequately informed about birth control. Problems of terminology, however, made it particularly difficult to find out precisely how much they know – problems our survey still leaves largely unsolved. If people do not understand the term 'birth control', does this imply that they are ignorant of contraceptives – or merely nonplussed by an unfamiliar phrase covering a familiar mechanism?

Knowledge

Although an easy majority of our sample seemed to understand the term 'birth control', one in twelve quite clearly did not know what it meant, one in twenty-five were wrong, [and] an additional fair-sized minority may or may not have understood. Out of every 100:

71 said birth control was limiting children
15 were very vague and may or may not have understood
8 frankly did not know
4 were wrong
and 2 refused to answer

The commonest misunderstanding arose from confusion of 'birth control' with the actual process of birth itself; the biggest group of those who were wrong though that it meant analgesia (head-line news at the time of the field-work on this survey) or some similar mechanism for assisting birth:

> *"It is a good idea, these new ideas of how to get children into the world without pain"* (24 year old bus service mechanic, St. Albans)

Some even disapprove of 'birth control' wrongly understood in this manner – an illustration of the way in which resistance to any idea may be based on verbal misapprehension:

> *"Well, I think it's made too easy for young girls these days, we used to suffer but we though it was worth it – now they can have children without any pain."* (60 year old wife of off-licensee's assistant, Battersea)

Occasionally, 'birth control' is confused with abortion – or even in a few cases understood as some sort of government regulation analogous to fuel control or rationing:

> *"I don't know, it's politics – one Government's as good as another, I think."* (50 year old unmarried housekeeper)

Ignorance and misunderstanding is most widespread amongst the unmarried; correspondingly the 25 – 44 year olds (the group presumably containing the highest proportion of sexually active marriages) has the clearest ideas about birth control. Women are worse informed than men – 5 women either do not know what birth control is or else confuse it with something else, to every three men. And an equally solid product of ignorance is the lowest educational group: 95% of all those who do not understand birth control have left school by the age of 14. The term 'birth control' seems to have no meaning for the following proportions in each educational group:

1% of those leaving school after $16\frac{1}{2}$
5% of those leaving school after 14 but not later than $16\frac{1}{2}$
14% of those leaving school up to 14

Similarly, only 2% of those earning over £10, and 26% of those earning less than £3 a week, are apparently ignorant of birth control. On the other hand knowledge seems to be little affected whether by town or country background (although people are slightly vaguer in country areas), neither is it affected by churchgoing nor religious habits. Equally, there is no apparent statistical relation between knowledge of birth control and attitudes to marriage and extra-marital relations. But it is difficult to make an exact quantitative assessment of knowledge on such a large scale as this; doubtful cases, doubtfully informed are sufficiently frequent to obscure group differences:

> *"I don't know, I never could fathom it ... I wouldn't have any."* (65 year old Old Age Pensioner (521))

> *"I wouldn't like to say much about it really, some use it, it might be all right."* (21 year old man, on demob leave (113))

Altogether probably about 80% of the adult population (16 years and over) have a roughly accurate idea of what birth control is. But ambiguities do not end here. Even granting some knowledge of birth control, it is difficult to know precisely what mechanisms people have in mind. Judging by the form taken by most replies, by no means everyone is thinking of contraceptives. Coitus interruptus seems generally to be regarded as a method of birth control, probably also the use of the safe period, possibly also in some cases abstention from intercourse. So far as it is possible for us to judge, the commonest interpretation is the use of contraceptives or withdrawal – although the latter is sometimes regarded as a more desirable alternative to 'birth control'. Very probably most people would not be able to say, even to themselves, precisely what they mean by birth control.

With such vague definitions in mind, the majority are in favour; out of every 100:

63 approve
15 disapprove
7 have mixed feelings
6 say they don't use contraceptives, or that they're too old
1 refuses to reply
8 don't know

Attitudes

For those whose feelings are so mixed that they refuse to come down on either side of the fence, birth control is often a two-edged weapon, potentially dangerous in the hands of the wrong people; these tend to stipulate that it should be used only in certain circumstances, usually reserving it for married people only:

> "Well, I don't know much about it, but when it's used by married people, I should say it's good." (22 year old woman, factory machinist, Bethnal Green)

> "I think it should only be used by those who cannot control themselves." (31 year old company secretary's wife, Fulham)

Others are just cautious, or perplexed:

> "There's a lot to be said for it, and a lot to be said against it ... it's to have a good time without the consequences." (26 year old postman (521))

Amongst those who know, more or less, what birth control is, men and women on the whole agree about its desirability. Marriage makes little difference; amongst the married group, parents and childless people again share similar attitudes except for more indecision on the part of those without children. Older church people are inclined to be more disapproving (70% of the under 34s approve, compared with 57% of those over 35). But the biggest difference occurs between the social classes. Approval increases with educational level, and particularly with income:

41% of those earning less than £3 a week approve of B.C.
65% of those earning up to £10 a week   "   "   "
71% of those earning over £10 a week   "   "   "

The financial cost of contraceptives may help to bias poorer people against them, but this aspect of the financial factor is very seldom mentioned; in any case, hostility to 'innovations' – particularly in the sexual field – is usually more common amongst the less well-off, and less adequately educated [....].

But opinion on birth control is usually affected by churchgoing habits and attitudes. 48% of all weekly churchgoers approve of birth control, compared with 68% of those who seldom or never go to church. Even excluding Roman Catholics, there is a 10% difference in figures of approval between churchgoers and non-churchgoers. But this difference of church attendance is partially a reflection of even more pronounced denominational influences (and it must be remembered that regular church goers are disproportionately Roman Catholic). Birth control is approved by:

64% of all Church of England churchgoers
64% of all Non-conformist churchgoers
37% of all Roman Catholic churchgoers

The difference in approval between present and past members of the Church of England (9%) is smaller than the difference between Church of England and Roman Catholic church-going groups (27%); it is clear that the influence of denomination on attitudes to birth control is stronger than the effect of churchgoing in itself. Moreover the early background of childhood churchgoing seems to have no perceptible influence at all; there is almost no difference in attitude between those people who were brought up in Church of England, Roman Catholic and Non-conformist churches, and who have since totally ceased to go to church. The all-important factor is the present denomination of active churchgoers.

Although the Catholic church is probably more hostile to birth control than any other institution in the present-day world, almost half of the Catholics in our sample were in favour of birth control methods. Moreover, these are by no means all renegade Catholics; about half of them had been to church within a week of answering our questions. At first sight this would seem to represent a large-scale repudiation of the Catholic church by its own members; but it must be remembered that some, at least, of this pro birth control Catholic group must be referring to the safe period (sanctioned by the Pope) – or even, like this 46 year old Catholic, to abstention from intercourse:

"If you love your wife enough not to burden her with a lot of children you must do it (practice birth control). When necessary birth control should be used. After you've got an agreed family fixed up between two people, it should be used. I don't mean artificial birth control methods, but when a family is big enough, a man must abstain." (46 year old advertiser's maintenance man, 117)

At what ever cost to himself, this man has established a religiously legitimate compromise between the demands of finance and of his Church. A great many Catholics, on the other hand, have quite frankly come into conflict with the teachings of a Church which they otherwise support; a practising Roman Catholic, for instance, who conforms to her Church's ethic on extra-marital relations, prostitution and divorce, says about birth control:

"Although it's against the Catholic religion, I thinks it's a worse sin to bring children up in want than to prevent them from coming." (55 year old railway clerk's wife, Nottingham, Roman Catholic)

As in this case, there is usually some suggestion of bad conscience where Catholics openly approve birth control; but the blame for the conflict is almost always placed on necessity, not on the Roman Catholic Church: but the guilty factors involved in this process make it at the very least possible that many more of those Catholics who explicitly rejected the principle of birth control, secretly approve it. Sometimes, for instance, opposition softens as confidence grows:

"Birth control is spacing children ... I don't like it on principle, but it is necessary for economic and selfish reasons" (32 year old wife of medical researcher, Roman Catholic)

But it is by no means always clear that Catholics realise the ambiguity of their situation when they approve of birth control. Some frankly discuss the conflict between their own viewpoint and that of the church, but many just register their approval, leaving their position as a church-goer [out] of account. Are they unaware of the Papal ruling? Or have they forced it to obscurity in the back of their mind? The latter suggestion seems the more likely one:

"The people who practise that are all more or less prostitutes."

But as the interviewer followed up on his views, this man began to show signs of conflicting feelings and to relax his opposition:

"It's a bit revolting. It depends more or less on the family. If it's not well off and can't support children, then I suppose it's all right."

And a factory foreman showed the same two-layer attitude:

> "I suppose it's money these days – there's no doubt about it. There's another big point, that the girls today don't want to be tied always in the home; they won't have it today. That's the reason, they don't want to be buggered about the kids – it's a fact ..."

But further questioning led to a climb down:

> "I do it myself, so I can't say anything against it." (54 year old foreman, Oxford, R.C.)

But sliding standards cannot always live peaceably side by side with continued allegiance to the Church. Sometimes the conflict between principle and practice becomes too great. A bookseller's assistant, for instance, who describes himself as:

> "I'm really a Roman Catholic, but I have my doubts."

and departs from his Church's ethic all along the line – divorce, extra-marital relations – is even enthusiastic over birth-control:

> "It's for the prevention of unwanted babies, and I should say it's an absolute social necessity. You'll not stop human nature – so why not control it scientifically in sex as in anything else?" (43 year old bookseller's assistant (232), Roman Catholic)

Nevertheless, the most bitter opposition to birth control comes from the Roman Catholic group:

> "That's a very wicked thing, you know. The Church doesn't allow it." (68 year old widow (441), R.C.)

> "It's to keep down the size of a family. But I don't believe in it – I believe it's a sin". (18 year old Junior in Bank (431), Roman Catholic)

For most Roman Catholics who still accept the Church's teaching on this point, judgement of birth control is made on entirely religious grounds. The fact that they are Catholic themselves is felt to be sufficient explanation of their attitude; very seldom is there any attempt at rationalising acceptance of the ruling; when this does occur it is usually along lines either of the selfishness [....] of those who use birth control, the artificiality of the method itself or the objection that contraception is a matter of taking lives. A middle aged railway inspector, Roman Catholic, takes the first view:

"I don't believe in it ... It's so as they can get out a bit, instead of being tied down."

Later in the interview, asked about the possible harmfulness of sex, this man replied – without apparently relating what he said to his earlier judgement on birth control:

"The only way I can think of is if you had a big family and your ways wouldn't allow you to keep them up."

A housewife, more orthodox, objects to birth control as murder:

"Well, I don't believe in it, being Roman Catholic. I don't believe in big families, but was never taught to believe in birth control – it's like taking a life, which is wrong." (27 year old fitter's wife, (231) R.C.)

But more regard the Church's teaching as [the] only justification necessary for their disapproval:

"It's against all our religious teachings, so I've never thought ... I have never interested myself in it, as it's against all my religious teachings." (32 year old surgeon's wife (113) R.C.)

"I don't study it because I'm R.C. I don't believe in it at all, you see I'm an R.C". (36 year old housewife)

Taken to its logical conclusion, Catholic adjustment to their Church's ruling against birth control properly ends in acceptance of the whole situation and all that it involves:

"Well, I couldn't say – I mean each one I've had I haven't grumbled, I've just had them and that's been that." (39 year old wife of Corporation Labourer (622), R.C.)

Religious conflict at a conscious level over the issue of birth control is largely confined, but not entirely, to Roman Catholics. Here, for instance, is a young man, no longer a Church-goer, but brought up as a Presbyterian:

"I don't see any purpose in it – its lack of purpose, children should be a purpose in life. It's really a sin against God in a way, but it's so difficult to raise a big family now." (Shipper's plater, aged 28, Greenock)

And a Church of England clergyman, interviewed non-professionally in the street[,] revealed similar conflicts:

"From the human stand point it's a good idea; from the Christian point of view it's wrong." (59 year old Minister (521))

Leading Opinion

Analysing the birth control attitude of our group of doctors, teachers and clergymen showed that:

84% of all doctors were in favour of birth control
78% of all teachers were in favour of birth control
49% of all clergymen "   "   "   "   "   "

The clergymen, almost all of whom belonged to the Church of England, were nearly as often mixed in their attitude as actually opposed to birth control. But mixed feelings in this case usually represent not perplexity, but more often the stipulation that contraceptives should not be used outside marriage; or except in cases of ill-health, for spacing, not eliminating, children. Almost none of this group – officially questioned as clergymen – reveal any [of the] conflict between principle and practice that troubles the man interviewed in the street. This 30 year old married clergyman is an exception:

"Absolutely, it is a perversion of the sex act. But in present economic conditions, it does prevent the misery of impossibly large families, and is therefore not to be finally condemned."

Apart from this recurrent proviso that contraceptives should be used only within marriage, or for spacing or health reasons, there is general approval of birth control amongst Church of England clergymen. Those who disapprove of it do so usually on moral rather than strictly religious grounds. The 1930 Lambeth Conference of Church of England Bishops resolved that, although abstention and self-discipline were to be preferred, other methods of birth control – unspecified – were permissible in certain cases of 'moral obligation'. This seems to be roughly the view of the clergymen – represented at this conference – who replied to our questionnaire. Not many condemn birth control as a sin; rather it is rejected as demoralising for those practising it, married or not; as immoral where it is used outside marriage; and as liable to encourage that sort of immorality. The emphasis is constantly placed on the need [for] restraint, self-discipline, abstention – *"self control, not birth control"*, as several describe it:

"It depends what you mean by it, I should like to forbid contraceptives, but I should not forbid self-restraint, practised without contraceptives." (62 year old Clergyman)

'Self-restraint' is an ambiguous terms; does it mean the practice of withdrawal, or – more drastically – does it recommend abstention? [....] But vaguely interpreted in this way, one clergyman in every four or five is entirely opposed to birth control; only one teacher in eight, on the other hand, and one doctor in thirteen, takes up a similar hostile attitude. Doctors, particularly, are inclined to consider the necessity of birth control from the more practical angles of health and finance, and as such approve. One young doctor, for instance:

> *"Modern financial conditions render it an essential part of family life*
> *– if we are to avoid great economic hardship in families, or an increase*
> *in illegal abortion and other un-natural methods of contraception.*
> *Modern contraception forms the least objectionable means to an end."*

A 40 year old G.P.:

> *"Birth control has always existed. The modern way of contraception*
> *is far better than the older methods of infanticide, exposure, etc. ......"*

A 43 year old surgeon describes his attitude briefly as "rational". And a doctor adds the warning:

> *"Birth control is infinitely preferable to withdrawal which is the cause*
> *of much neurosis."*

Teachers take up much the same position, except that they are rather less inclined to judge the matter on practical grounds and slightly more apt to condemn it from the moral-religious view-point. A 46 year old Catholic teacher, for instance, gives the religiously orthodox answer:

> *"I am all in favour of 'self-control'. Birth control, and extra-marital*
> *intercourse, pre-marital intercourse and divorce all pander to the*
> *weak-willed and self-indulgent who are, after all, not worthy mem-*
> *bers of society."*

About equally favourable to birth-control, with doctors and teachers, were members of Mass-Observation's National Panel. Only 3% of this group condemn it outright, and four out of every five are unreservedly in favour – mostly on grounds of economic necessity and the undesirability of having 'too many' children. Moreover, detailed questioning about their sex habits showed that only one tenth of the married couples represented in this group used no form of birth control at all – and in half of these cases, one partner was infertile. Where birth control was used, mechanical and chemical contraceptives were far commoner than the other methods such as the safe period (note 1). In their attitudes, members of this group seem to take up the position of the more 'progressive' ranks of the middle class. Except for the proviso, from about one in ten, that use of contraceptives should be reserved for married people, birth control is accepted more or less as a matter of course – as necessary and desirable within the set-up of present day conditions:

> *"Life would be hell without it. Either frustration or an incomplete relationship with one's husband, and consequent bickering." (35 year old housewife)*

With a few objections from Roman Catholics, and an occasional hesitation on the score of immorality, [....] selfishness, and nervous ill-effects, so-called 'educated' opinion is whole-heartedly in favour of birth control, and less educated opinion does not seem to be far behind.

Motives

Just over a quarter of those of the street sample who approve of birth control give no reason for their attitude – they simply say that it is a good thing and leave it at that. To many of these, as to even more of the Panel group with their higher educational background, birth control would seem to be something to be taken more or less for granted – not only necessary but also often with very positive and beneficial qualities of its own:

> *"Birth control is to enable you to live a full life, and not to have children unless you want them. It's an excellent thing."* (34 year old draughtsman (232))

The Panel group is especially prone to emphasise the positive benefits of birth control, rather than the purely negative aspect of prevention alone. An elderly woman, for instance:

> *"It is designed for economic and essential happiness."*

> *"I'm not exactly against it, because of the cost of living, but in normal times it's natural to want a large family."* (46 year old woman, housekeeping for brother, Bethnal Green)

Sometimes, but less often, the emphasis shifts beyond the apologetic note to the more positive feeling that birth control is a necessary evil made meritable only by inadequate incomes:

> *"Money! That's the only purpose of it. A wee income and you can't afford anything but a wee family. I don't really hold with it. A man's wage should be big enough to bring up a family."* (74 year old OAP, Glasgow)

Only occasionally, at the other extreme, and amongst the very poorest groups, do a few people feel that this phase of economic necessity is passing, and that Family Allowances have turned children into a financial asset:

> *"Well, birth control is all right, if you haven't the money to keep them with. But it is to your advantage to have children now that you get 5/- a week each for them."* (53 year old widow, Manchester)

But for most people, birth control is a financial necessity, and as such is accepted in a matter of fact and more or less circumstantial manner. Closely interlinked with this money argument is the feeling expressed by one in three of those in favour of birth control – that the smaller-sized, deliberately spaced family is in all ways the most desirable. This group is more firmly convinced a few children are almost always preferable to many; on the other hand, very few of them – and very few of any of those who approve of birth control – regard contraception as a means of having no children at all:

> *"It should be used to space your family. Too many don't give the others a chance. I think it's a very good thing; to have too many isn't fair to the mother or to the rest."* (47 year old policeman's wife, York)

> *"I naturally use birth control – I definitely feel one should for the purpose of planning the family, not to prevent having children."* (35 year old commercial traveller's wife, St. Albans)

For a few, the smaller family is additionally preferable in that it leaves the wife relatively free to pursue her own interests as an individual, rather than a machine for producing unwieldy families:

> *"Well I think this – that wives have so much to think about these days, and so much to do; and they are tied in so many ways if they have large families; I think a wife should have some interests outside the home."* (46 year old agricultural worker's wife, Oxford)

Other reasons for favouring birth control are mentioned much less often. Health and housing came up to a roughly equal extent from both sexes, and with little difference between age or class groups; health reasons usually have the mother in mind – the ill-health and fatigue that may either result from too frequent pregnancies or render childbearing undesirable in the first place:

> *"I think it (birth control) should be in some cases. There's a poor woman near me has one every year, she's expecting one now and I bet you in ten months there'll be another."* (48 year old woman telephonist, Westminster)

Housing difficulties represent a problem of which most people have had at least second-hand experience; many say that this is why they have had to use birth control themselves:

> *"You must have birth control. My wife and I would very much like to have a family, but we haven't got a house, and you can't have a family in someone else's house."* (29 year old P.O. engineer, Newcastle)

Even a middle-aged Roman Catholic, who said *"I've buried five, but I don't believe in birth control"*, could see the force of the housing argument:

> *"People just getting married won't have children because there's a lot of these landladies who won't take couples in because they have children ... If there were more houses there's be more children."*

The minority who bring up population reasons to support their approval of birth control are chiefly men; women are, as usual, more involved with the more personal and practical aspects of the matter. This 55 year old (441) farmer speaks with middle-aged experience and conviction:

> *"It's to keep down families. I agree with it. It's no good breeding like animals, over-populating the world, letting people come into the world to have them starve of hunger."*

When women consider birth control in its wider setting of society and the world in general, they are often, even then, still focusing on the individual; with wars and starvation, the world of today is no fit place to bear children into. One London housewife, for instance:

> *"I agree with birth control. I had three boys. At 18 they went into the Army. I wouldn't have had any if I had known."*

Generally, people have accepted birth control neither with enthusiasm nor with resignation, but purely as a practical inevitability. For a minority, on the other hand, it remains a concession to present day conditions. To some extent this semi-reluctance may be a matter of mollifying the vague stirrings of a guilty morality, and to some extent it may also represent a genuine wistfulness for large unplanned families; but to most people the inconveniences of the large family are only too painfully clear (note 2). A few go so far as to discuss birth control vaguely as a symptom of a new outlook; references to changed ideas, increasing freedom, favourable comparisons with the families of Victorian days, creep in from time to time. For a minority – particularly the younger and more educated minority – birth control seems to confer new and positive blessings of its own:

> *"Well, nobody wants their wife to go on having children year after*

year like they used to – things are different now. I don't want more than two or three at the most – couldn't afford them apart from anything else." (27 year old road-mender, Oxford)

But enthusiasm over birth control is a minority attitude. For some – equally a minority – it is definitely undesirable, to those looking at the other side of the picture, white becomes black, expediency turns into foolishness, [....] immorality and even sin.

No Opposition

The minority who disapprove of birth control are even less inclined to explain their motives than those who approve. Half of them, particularly women, say it is wrong or undesirable, and give no specific reason, probably because this group consists disproportionately of churchgoers, particularly Catholics, thinking largely in terms of absolute morality that does not need explanation. Amongst those who go more deeply into their attitudes, the most common objections are that birth control is un-natural, religiously wrong[....]. But of every hundred of those disapproving:

51 just said birth control was wrong or undesirable
15 said it was unnatural
12 expressed religious objections
12 said it was a sign of or conducive to [.....]
6   objected on political or population grounds
2   said it was a sign or, or conducive to immorality
1   said it had psychological effects
1   said it was inefficient or ineffective
3   made miscellaneous objections
(some objected for more than one type of reason)

Religious objections, most frequent amongst women, have already been discussed. Men are more inclined to object to birth control because they feel it to be unnatural.

This resistance to birth control as an artificial mechanism has these stages of development: first, that children, not contraceptives, are 'natural'; second, that to 'go against nature' is bad in itself; and third, that to do so will cause actual harm to the transgressor. Here are the first two stages:

"well, some people don't like children, so they don't have them. But that's not human, it's not nature, I mean trees have to grow little trees and dogs have to have puppies." (47 year old wife of unemployed (111) man)

"I can't understand that (using birth control). What do they want to

> get married for? They just want to have a good time. I wouldn't like
> to be on that game. If children come, let them come." (67 year old
> pensioner, Newcastle)

Less often this attitude is extended to the belief that contraceptives may do
bodily or psychological harm, or even possibly cause infertility. Occasionally,
the use of birth control is confused with childlessness, leaving clear the objection that women will suffer physically in the end if they have no children at all:

> "Well I don't know. They (childless women) get tumours and die, and
> that. I had a lovely friend die because she hadn't had any." (65 year
> old Policeman's widow, Westminster)

> "It isn't good for the health, not all them contraceptives ain't" (36
> year old welder's wife, Manchester)

In a later more comprehensive survey it would be profitable to follow up
these hints and warnings, to discover how far they are based on experience,
how far they have a traditional basis, and how far they represent spontaneous
individual attempts to rationalise what is felt to be wrong and unnatural. It
would be equally interesting to trace back the viewpoint of those who condemn birth control as something used only by the [lazy] and selfish and
degenerate:

> "It's for human lust. I can't see any other reason for it." (30 year old
> chemist's assistant, Hendon)

> "It's all right for a lazy woman, they don't want to be bothered." (71
> year old pensioner, Glasgow)

> "I think women is very cheap if they allow that." (56 year old stew-
> ard in Merchant Service, Edinburgh)

> "I never had anything to do with it. I had eight children. It never both-
> ered me. Four were killed in the war and two died, but I never had
> anything to do with birth control. It's a modern idea, they don't want
> to bring up families, – they want a good time." (83 year old pension-
> er, Ayr)

Only a very few reject birth control on the more practical grounds that it is
ineffective. This man is unusual:

> "I've never had any use for it. It lets you down, anyway." (71 year old
> retired soldier, Oxford)

And an extract from the sex case history of a young working class

woman show a similarly rarely expressed scepticism:
"I was worried about that (having intercourse with a man friend) and thought I was going to have a baby, and I told him so. He told me that he wore a sort of rubber glove, and that while he had that on I could-n't have a baby. At the time I though that you had a baby just with 'going' with a man, whether you wore anything or not. I didn't believe him, I did not have any more to do with him."

Fear of pregnancy, and presumably distrust or ignorance of contraceptives, is clearly an important factor in discouraging pre-marital relations. Of our National Panel group, one in every six mentioned this as a reason for refraining from sex relations with their husband or wife before marriage. Even so, fear of pregnancy was mentioned less frequently by this groups than either moral objections, or – more vaguely – simply that they 'did not want to' (presumably a largely moral attitude). More widespread knowledge of efficient methods of contraception would certainly influence some in the direction of unsanctioned sex relations, [although] fear of pregnancy seems to be by no means the main factor involved.

Resistance to birth control does not take an entirely negative form. Some of those who approve of it think wistfully of the joys of the large family, and in the same way disapproval is sometimes based on the feeling that children are such a blessing that one should not want to prevent them. Once again the objection is a logically irrelevant one, in as much as it is often based on a confusion of contraception with total childlessness, an association which is much more common amongst those who disapprove of birth control than amongst those who accept it. But most people's ideas are vague and often confused, and when it comes to building up attitudes, irrelevant reasons are at heart equally powerful and important with the more strictly logical ones. Even so it is difficult to tell how deep seated, how merely a matter of lip-service to convention, is this vaguely suggestive enthusiasm for the large family as a special source of happiness. Certainly most people are sufficiently aware to put it into its financial context, and its usual form is merely to regard birth control as a vaguely inferior alternative to the large family. But there is an example of the less cautious exponents of this view:

"There's a good many who don't want children. They are fools to themselves. They have no one to think for, no one to see them in their old age. I've met men that way. There's always more happiness when there's a house full of children coming along." (72 year old retired miner, now a builder's labourer, Stafford)

And a Chester undertaker, ex-publican, sums it up:

"Marriage without children is like a garden without flowers."

Opposition to birth control, although a minority attitude, retains a virility that no doubt derives from its religious – particularly Catholic – background [....]. Birth control still seems to be a focus for personal and individual conflicts at varying levels of consciousness; it is not necessary to dig very deep to discover morality at war with expediency, instilling a sense of uneasiness with the arguments on either side.

Notes

1 Detailed results of the birth control habits of this group will be found in Appendix 1.
2 Apart from the evidence of this survey, the 1945 M-O investigation of the reasons behind the falling birth rate, making a direct approach to the problem of size of family, concluded that *"By far the most popular family size is two children, which three out of every five of newly married couples would like. The proportion who would like more than three children declining rapidly down the scale of length of marriage, and only 8% of those married less than five years want as many as this."* Britain and her Birth-Rate, published John Murray, 1945.

Chapter Five: Marriage

Whatever the manners of the past, present-day customs tend publicly to two contrary attitudes to marriage; the romantic and sentimental approach of the novelist, and the practical jeers of the music hall comedian concentrating on the nagging wife, messy baby, and interfering mother-in-law. In the background, well away from the lime-light, the Church discusses marriage from its spiritual and religious stand-point, and even more remotely the biologist and moralist quietly point out the relation of marriage to sex. Somewhere in the middle, the 'man in the street' has developed his own conception of marriage, to some extent a compromise but relatively free of the perplexity that might be expected to result from a variety of conflicting influences, To the ordinary man, marriage is an entirely desirable and practical institution – so long as it is approached with caution; it is difficult to discover much sentiment or romanticism in his opinion, and almost equally it is wrong to accuse him of the exaggerated disillusionment that is so popular with music halls.

Asked how they felt about marriage, just over half of our street sample approved of it unreservedly; of the remainder most were not un-favourable, but merely guarded; out of every 100:

58   were unreservedly in favour of marriage
15   were in favour provided the partners were cautious and co-operated
8   said it depended on the people
5   said it depended on material facts – housing, money etc.
4   had mixed feelings
4   gave unfavourable opinions
4   did not know or were vague
2   made miscellaneous comments

This question was regarded by Mass-Observation investigators as a 'safe question' – one which could generally be relied upon to be received with interest and without the embarrassment or resentment that some of the later questions on more specifically sexual subjects sometimes aroused. People enjoyed discussion on marriage – it is a subject of which most of them had personal experience and almost everyone had thought about this. Moreover, this very interest and first-hand personal acquaintance with marriage also meant that they were the better able to judge the matter for themselves, and less inclined to give the conventional reply. Mass-Observation has found in other surveys that the nearer the topic under discussion approaches to people's own lives, the more their opinion tends to be moulded by their own personal experience, rather than by what they imagine other – more important – people think; where a prominent opinion with which they have morally found themselves in sympathy conflicts with their own personal ideas and experiences, the result tends to be perplexity – the [previous] chapter, for instance, revealed the indecisive state in which many Roman Catholics now find themselves on birth control (note 1). But in the case of marriage people are more inclined to feel themselves on firm ground.

It is this close personal experience of marriage that enables so many people to see it free of romance and glamour and involves them in the expression of opinions with a very different emphasis to that of the 'expert' groups – which we questioned less as individuals and more as representatives of their professions; doctors, teachers and clergymen. Of these, out of every 100:

90 clergymen were unreservedly in favour of marriage
80 teachers "   "   "   "   "   "   "
70 doctors "   "   "   "   "   "   "

To clergymen, questioned as clergymen, marriage tends to be a spiritual undertaking, essentially desirable in itself; only one in seventeen ever mentions the necessity for caution before marrying and, once married, for co-operation between partners:

> *"It is a holy vocation"* (56 year old clergyman)

> *"It should be on the highest plane revealed to us, and according to the Marriage Service of the Church of England, only so can we assist our children in the greatest battle of their lives and raise the tone of family life generally."* (72 year old missionary)

But most clergymen put the emphasis not only on the sanctity of marriage, but also on its permanency, an angle that is less clearly in the forefront of the layman's mind:

> *"Marriage is a holy state – an indissoluble union of one man and one woman, till death parts them!"* (48 year old clergyman)

Only a minority of the clergymen who answered our questionnaire envisage marriage in a less exalted and perfectionist light:

"I am convinced that the classic Christian view of the 'sanctity' of marriage should be upheld as being the best view there is. But there needs to be more sympathy and help given to those whose marriages fall short of the Christian standards". (45 year old vicar)

Teachers see marriage on a rather lower plane; but even they show a tendency to emphasise the religious sanctity and permanency of marriage as well as to conceive it in broad terms as the necessary and inevitable basis of human life. But they are a little more willing than the clergymen group to take into account human weakness and failings:

"Marriage is a life-long mission between two people who love each other; through constant companionship, tolerance and comforting they may achieve life-long happiness and a life more worth-while living than a life lived on one's own. But effort is required." (26 year old schoolmaster.)

"I regard it as a necessity fundamental for our society. I hold the view that no sexual intercourse should take place without its blessing, but I realise that this latter view is an ideal rather than a practical state of affairs." (24 year old schoolmaster)

A few teachers – with the children in mind – see marriage from a partly educational point of view:

"I think that two people contemplating marriage should regard it as a means by which they can live a full life in happy companionship and provide for their children in an atmosphere of love and security." (48 year old schoolmaster)

On the whole, teachers as a group differ from the people interviewed in the street chiefly in that they place more emphasis on the wider social values of marriage as well as on its religious aspects – and are rather less inclined to think of the practical difficulties that it may involve. Doctors, too, show much the same pattern, except for an occasional medical bias:

"Marriage is a psycho-physical relationship depending for its success on a perfect harmony both in the mental and physical aspects. Maladjustments of either causes unhappiness in proportion to the degree of imbalance." (39 year old doctor)

In these groups, references to the sex factor in marriage are almost equally rare with any mention of the more material factors of housing or finance. Few replies emphasise anything but the social and emotional value of marriage both to society and the individual, its sanctity and permanence and – where warnings are given – the need for caution in choosing partners, and for long and full co-operation once marriage has begun. Almost all are couched in a long range, very different to that of the man interviewed in the street; very few for instance reply as simply and directly as this 32 year old doctor:

"I'm married anyway. It's a good thing."

[....These] groups of doctors, teachers and clergymen are probably surveyed in the direction of conventionality by the fact that they were interviewed to some extent as representatives of their professions. Members of Mass-Observation's National Panel, very roughly a comparable middle class group, although on a rather lower professional level, were asked for their views as individuals, quite irrespective of their job or profession. Perhaps partly a reflection of this more anonymous and personal approach, perhaps also because the Panel is more Left-Wing and less religiously inclined – as well as on the whole considerably younger than the groups of doctors, teachers and clergymen – members of the National Panel tend to give much less conventional views, and are less inclined to think of marriage in terms of sanctity and the spirit. Except that they see it more often from a wider social point of view, marriage appears to the Panel in much the same light as it appears to the 'man in the street', and about the same proportion approve it unreservedly; to them it is a personal arrangement, at its best productive of much happiness and stability, but necessitating caution, co-operation and mutual adjustment if an equal degree of unhappiness and instability is to be avoided:

"I want to get married. I should put everything I have into making my marriage a very happy one. I should treat that as being far more important than anything else." (22 year old journalist, Panel member)

"Marriage is essential for a full and happy life." (39 year old RAF engineering officer, Panel member)

"Very seldom a success, but worth trying." (39 year old export manager, Panel member)

"As an institution I am all for it for those whom it suits – which is the majority. I have no belief in its divine origin or with sanctity per se." (38 year old estate agent)

This grocer member of the Panel takes the practical-causal view of marriage to its extreme degree:

"It does not seem to me that I had any particular feelings about my marriage apart from the desire to get married to a particular person.

I remember I tried to avoid all fuss. It was much against my will that I had to have a peculiar ceremony in a particular building in which a man wearing his collar back to front gave me permission to go and live with my wife. He added, I believe, some entirely gratu- itous advice about being fruitful which seemed to me indelicate and purely a matter for my own personal decision. Later we found that the parson had validated our marriage without being in possession of a requisite document, so a parson came and took the certificate away for some reason. It never came back. I mentioned to my sister in law that apparently my wife and I had been living in sin for some months and she was horrified, saying 'The marriage was bad enough and now this'. However all was well as we were able to obtain another cer- tificate without difficulty."

Even the sex factor in marriage occasionally creeps into the replies of some of this group:

"Though I cannot think that a man, at any rate, is naturally monoga- mous, in society as at present constituted marriage provides a reason- able fair solution to the problem of sex first – but also of the neces- sary developments, or limitations of one's personality." (35 year old schoolmaster, Panel member)

Perhaps much of the difference between this group and the more admonitory attitude of the doctors, teachers and clergymen is summed up by this 45 year old physicist:

"Marriage is more like the Song of Solomon than the injunctions of Paul!"

To 'the man in the street', even more than the Panel Group, marriage is nei- ther a spiritual nor moral, but purely mundane personal arrangement designed for people's comfort and happiness – an arrangement, however, which is easily capable of going wrong. Marriage for them is wholly desirable provided the partners are suitable and capable of mutual adjustment, and provided material difficulties are not too great. Their views are halfway between the romantic conception of marriage and the paradox of the music hall. They see marriage as studded with pitfalls for the unwary, and, con- versely, as an entirely practical and individual affair that at best can provide intense emotional satisfaction for those who manage it well. But almost no one regards it as an automatic road to happiness:

"Well, if it wasn't for the money – I only feel it's hard just now. It all goes on food, you've got nothing over for clothes or anything for the house. I'm quite contented the other way. It's better since we lived out

> *here and had a garden again – for a good time we lived in Hattwhistle and we hadn't got one. I work it out a garden saves you near 10/- a week on vegetables."* (37 year old wife of factory labourer, Hattwhistle)

> *"It's a good thing if you fall in love with the right partner."* (34 year old unemployed farm labourer)

And this middle aged wife of a Yorkshire joiner feels that married happiness is something that you only have with time:

> *"Well, you grow into it. You get used to it. The first ten years you spend getting used to it, the next ten you are used to it, the last ten you begin to reap the reward."*

'Ifs' and 'buts' come into the views on marriage of one in every three of the street sample. The most frequent qualification mentioned by one in every seven is made in terms of the necessity for caution in getting married, and, particularly, the need for give and take between husband and wife:

> *"It's fine if you pull together."* (45 year old bus driver's wife, 632)

> *"It has its ups and downs like everything else. I should say you get out of it according to what you put into it."* (47 year old widow, dentist's receptionist.)

> *"It's the best thing in life if you both pull the same way."* (36 year old marine fitter's wife, 721)

One in thirteen stresses the importance of choosing the right partner:

> *"It's all right. A good wife is just as good as your mother, if she's a good wife."* (73 year old OAP, Greenock)

> *"It's all right with the right sort of partner, if not it's rotten."* (50 year old wife of fish and chip shop proprietor, Reading)

And one in twenty insists that a successful marriage depends on its material assets:

> *"It's good enough if you can get the man that will keep you. If you are going to be poor, you might just as well be poor by yourself."* (50 year old Canteen worker, Hendon)

> *"If I had a home it would be wonderful. As it is we're separated, and I've been married in name only for the past three years."* (33 year old carpenter's wife, Bethnal Green)

'Ifs' and 'buts' apart, however, the 'man in the street' is very much in favour of marriage – even if he usually sees it largely devoid of glamour or romance. He is by no means over-enthusiastic, but generally speaking regards marriage as a 'fine thing' and the best 'natural' way of living. For the most part it is only in this latter oblique way that the sex factor in marriage is referred to:

> *"It's the only institution there is."* (42 year old wife of elect[rical] engineer, 663)

> *"It's the natural state for all men and women to be in."* (46 year old policeman's wife.)

> *"I don't think a fellow can go through life without marrying and enjoying himself."* (48 year old Engineering Machinist, 522)

Enthusiasm, when it occurs, usually has a personal bearing:

> *"If everyone has the same wife as I've got, the world would go round champion."* (62 year old docker, Newcastle)

> *"I'm happily married. It's a wonderful life to me."* (48 year old civil servant's wife, 634)

Men and women seem to think more or less alike on the subject of marriage, but enthusiasm increases slightly in proportion to the frequency with which people go to church; more pronouncedly favourable feelings go down with declining level in the social scale. 61% of all middle class people are whole-heartedly in favour of marriage (a frequency of unreserved approval higher than that of any other group we investigated), compared with 57% of the artisan and 51% of people with unskilled working class backgrounds. The lower people's social level, the more lukewarm and sceptical they tend to get about marriage, and the more inclined to stress the need for caution and co-operation. Even more influential is the question of whether people are married themselves. Unmarried people are less inclined to commit themselves to an opinion of marriage, but when they do pass an opinion it is less often a favourable one. 58% of our married group are more or less whole-heartedly in favour of marriage, compared with only 41% of the unmarried – and, in addition, more of the married group [are] in favour of marriage provided there is co-operation between partners. Single people are not so much hostile to marriage as cautious; they are particularly inclined to insist on the importance of material factors such as housing and finance, as well as the need for choosing partners, and for co-operation, having chosen them. Least enthusiastic, and more cautious of any group, about marriage are unmarried people over 30; only 34% of this group approve of marriage without reservation.

But only very few people are really against marriage: even in the unmarried over 30 group only 6% give entirely unfavourable opinions. Those who do disapprove are usually either disillusioned about their own experience, or else regard marriage as something not for them. An OAP from York, for instance, has long since given up the idea:

> "I got jilted in the first war, and I haven't bothered since."

And a labourer, cryptically:

> "I was going to get married, but I had a bit of bother with her auntie."
> (29 year old labourer, Chester)

A wife, embittered by an undomesticated husband:

> "Well, men are very selfish, they ought to wash up – my husband is lazy – put that down. I work 8.30 to 6.30 and do everything in the house." (45 year old shop assistant, factory worker's wife. 113)

A young Bristol office clerk feels that present day housing conditions rule out marriage entirely as far as he is concerned:

> "Personally I've no interest in it as conditions are now. If you get married you've got to live with your parents."

And a widower of 30 years standing, regards marriage as too ambitious an undertaking:

> "St. Paul never married, nor St. Peter, nor Christ. And Christ said there are no marriages in heaven. I find that the fact of being bound to one person all your life makes it possible for so many things to upset the harmony. I haven't a good thing to say for marriage." (90 year old retired teacher, Manchester)

Significantly, or not, this man found out about sex in the following way:

> "You come across companions with funny photographs, and they tell you funny tales, and gradually you get inquisitive and begin to ask questions."

The anti-married minority is a hybrid group, best considered in relation to the background of the individuals composing it. Often their hostility to marriage is quite consistent, not only with the rest of their attitude, but also with what we were able to discover of their personal history. One disillusioned Manchester wife of a wagon builder, for instance, herself a machinist, 45 years old and with two grown up children, says about marriage:

"If I had my time over again, I don't think I would get married at all."

This woman had an unhappy home background, disliking her father (*"a man expects too much of a woman, and he did from her"*); she received no useful sex instruction (*"I didn't find out about things until it was too late"*), does not believe that sex is necessary for happiness (*"That's a man's version of it, but I don't think it's the same with a woman"*), resents her husband's sexual demands (*"I think I do quite all right, I don't let him go short, but I think a man wants too much of it"*), and believes that sex *"can be cheap"*. All in all the pattern is rounded and complete.

An easy going 52 year old Hattwhistle unmarried labourer seems consistently – and insistently – uninterested in sex, and unemotional about all its aspects:

"I was disappointed in life years ago, and I've never bothered since about marriage .... some can go through a full life and never think nothing about sex, but they're very very few. I have done."

An Oxford labourer's wife, 46 years old, with two children, disillusioned about marriage (*"If I'd known what it was going to be like I wouldn't have married"*), found out about sex "from friends". She considers extra-marital relations and prostitution as *"disgusting" and* "has no time for" divorce; about sex, she says:

"To tell you the truth, I think it is very unpleasant. My husband says I'm not human. If I'd known what it was like before I got married I would never have married."

The investigator felt that this woman was subnormal mentally, her attitudes form a consistent pattern, but we have no indications at all of why they took this shape. This Edinburgh OAP, on the other hand, with an apparently normal attitude to sex is unmarried even though 68 (*"My race is run, I'm 68"*) and has his reason, however superficial, ready to hand:

"My father was a plasterer, and when he was alive trade was a washout, he couldn't make a living – and that's what made me what I was. I decided I was not going to ask a woman to go through what my mother had to contend with."

Sometimes it is possible to get some sort of understanding of people's attitudes to marriage, in light of the general set-up of their other attitudes and background; but it is dangerous to generalise on a basis of brief case-history impressions alone. Statistical evidence, however, allows an opportunity for less easily controvertible generalisations; and this may be provided by correlating attitudes to marriage with other factors, Results show that people who condemn extra-marital relations are – understandably – most inclined to favour marriage (7% difference between the two groups, but this is largely a matter of married disapproval of unorthodox sex relations); that people who say that generally it is impossible to be happy without some form of sex life are also most in favour of marriage (but again this to some extent reflects the difference between marriage and single (6% difference)); and that people who seem most contented (who are most inclined to say that they are getting what they want from life, an attitude no more frequent amongst married than single) are also most inclined to approve marriage unreservedly (11% difference). In other words, whole-hearted approval of marriage seems to be to some extent an attitude of the more contented and the more well-adjusted; but again there is no way of discovering whether the contentment and adjustment are a cause or an effect of pro-marriage feeling. Similarly, unmarried people over 30 – the 'confirmed' bachelor group – are a little more inclined than the group as a whole to distrust sex as possibly unpleasant; is this a matter of 'sour grapes'? Or is this one reason why, consciously or unconsciously, they have so far avoided marriage? But our results also suggest that a background of unhappily married parents is liable to make people sceptical of marriage themselves. 56% of those with happily married parents were unreservedly in favour of marriage, compared with 45% of those who admitted that their parents' marriage was not successful (note 2). An unhappy parental example seems to incline people not so much towards anti-marriage feeling, as towards reservations and wariness – insistence on suitable partners, the need for co-operation, and so on.

The success or failure of the parents' married life quite clearly exercises more influence on their children's developing attitude to marriage. Additional evidence of this is the fact that unmarried people over thirty (the group selected as probably containing the highest proportion of people predisposed against marriage, unconsciously or otherwise) are slightly less inclined than the total sample to claim a background of happily married parents. An unhappy parental background seems not only to produce anti-marriage feeling, but may also put that feeling into practice by maintaining bachelorhood.

If the early family background provided by parents' marital relations has so important an influence on the later attitudes of the children to marriage, what is it that is most frequently mentioned as going wrong? Three-quarters of our whole sample claimed a happy married life for their parents, so that proportions admitting each type of failure are very small. Out of every 100 of the entire 2,052 interviewed:

4   said their parents' marriage was spoilt by drink
3   said their parents were unsuited, or quarrelled
3   said one or both parents died when they were still young
2   said the marriage was spoilt by poverty
2   said the marriage was spoilt by the father's behaviour

1   "   "   "   "   " ill-health
1   said the parents separated or were divorced
1   said there were too many children
1   said the marriage was unsatisfactory, for unknown reasons

But drink would seem to be a declining factor in upsetting marriages; it is mentioned chiefly by the over 45s. This 30 year old woman is an exception:

> *"No, they didn't have a happy married life together, my father used to drink a terrible lot, always coming back full of beer he was."* (30 year old labourer's wife, Hendon)

Appendix 1 of this report, discussing the sex habits of the National Panel group, gives details of attempts to correlate early family background with present marital adjustment. These correlations mostly drew a blank, but the results, though negative, are intensely interesting. The Panel group was asked, amongst other background questions, whether they came into conflict with their parents, whether their mother was 'very clean and tidy', and what was their parents' attitude to sex. Perhaps attempts to isolate single factors as determinant of complex attitudes are inevitably doomed to failure; each of these produced entirely negative results.

Finally, as a conclusion to a chapter mainly devoted to discussing attitudes to marriage, it may be interesting to add a note on habit. Most people, it has been seen, have a more or less realistic and mundane view of marriage [....], not noticeably inclining towards either the romanticism of literature or the jeers of the music hall – and to all intents and purposes quite alien to the more spiritual view of the Church. Attitudes expressed by the Mass-Observation Panel group were very similar to those of the street sample. Although this group was a little more inclined to raise marriage from a personal to a social function, their outlook was still largely devoid of spirituality, romanticism, or excessive cynicism. Panel divulgence of the fact of their sex life and marital adjustment is particularly interesting in that it helps to reveal the behaviour cloaked by the verbal attitude.

Three-quarters of the Panel group, as Appendix 1 shows in more detail, said that they were satisfied – often very satisfied – with their married lives; only one in twenty was definitely unsatisfied. 82% of all the men were completely satisfied by marital intercourse, and 61% of the women – a striking difference between sexes. Exactly half the women of this group said that they usually or always experienced an orgasm; women are clearly much worse off than men in this respect. Correlations show that sexual satisfaction is very closely related to marital happiness, and perhaps this is one reason why so many people continuously insist on the need for carefully chosen partners, full co-operation and mutual adjustment. It may be no coincidence that the improvement most often desired for making marital sexual relationships more satisfactory was increased co-operation and responsiveness in lovemaking on the part of the husband or wife.

Finally, neither Panel nor Street opinions of marriage often mention the need for complete sexual fidelity – although no doubt this is often implied. But even though extra-marital relations in the Panel group were less frequently admitted than sex relations before marriage, they are still acknowledged by one husband in every four and one wife in every five. At first sight, sexual fidelity would seem to be no vital factor in marital adjustment; but it is significant that extra-marital intercourse is closely connected with unhappiness in marriage – although there is no way of knowing whether this is a cause of the unhappiness or result of it; one in five of the happily married has experienced an extra-marital affair, compared with one in three of the unhappy. It is possible to be satisfied with marriage without entire sexual fidelity, even though the norm of the happy marriage would seem to be monogamy (post-maritally at least). Perhaps it is because most husbands and wives are sexually faithful to their partners that so few feel the need to emphasise the necessity for fidelity when discussing their attitudes to marriage.

Notes

1 Another example of the process refers back to newspaper comment on the parliamentary issue of suspending the death penalty. Working class origin and Right-wing politics were the decisive factors producing opinion favouring the Suspension. The *Daily Mirror*, read largely by Labour working class readers, was editorially in favour of retaining the death penalty. The result was a high degree of 'don't know, perplexed' opinion amongst *Daily Mirror* readers (see *The Press and its Readers* by Mass-Observation).
2 Naturally, many may have been impelled by prestige moves falsely to claim that their parents marriage was a happy one. Also admission of an unsuccessful parental marriage may be the result, not the cause, of anti-marriage feelings. Our results can give only a rough suggestion of probably determining factors.

Chapter Six: Divorce

Statistics show that one marriage gets dissolved each year for every nine that take place. Most people have at least second-hand experience of divorce; and many more know at first hand the unsatisfactory conditions from which a divorce may spring. Like marriage, and unlike – for instance – prostitution, divorce is a subject on which ordinary men and women may be expected to make up their own minds, their opinions only partially determined by what other more important-seeming people say.

On the subject of marriage, the 'man in the street', together with our Panel group of middle class 'progressives', showed himself reluctant whole-heartedly to adopt the enthusiastic attitude of medical, educational and religious opinion; on sex education he tagged along in the wake of the professional groups; on birth control he was unhappily caught between the opposing forces of Church and the lay professions. And comparison of the views of each group on the subject of divorce gives much the same results for birth control. Doctors, teachers and Panel group line up together with the highest rate of approval, vacillating half way down the scale in the street sample representing the opinion of the whole population, and least favourably of all, are the clergymen.

In each group, out of every hundred:

83 of the Panel group more or less approve of divorce
75 of the Doctors "   "   "   "   "   "
70 of the teachers "   "   "   "   "   "
57 of the street sample   "   "   "   "   "
33 of the clergymen   "   "   "   "   "

For most clergymen the main issue is not simply one of divorce, but divorce with remarriage – a distinction that occurs much less often amongst street sample views. Seeing marriage in religious terms of sanctity and permanency, it becomes permissible in certain cases, notably adultery, to divorce or separate; but only a few condone remarriage afterwards.

> *"Divorce may be essential if the parties are quite hopelessly unsuitable or even if one of them is – But no marriage after it."* (47 year old school chaplain)

A minority of clergymen make an exception of non-church goers; but again this distinction is confined almost entirely to themselves:

> *"For believers in Christ it is forbidden. For others it should be discouraged, except in cases of great hardship."* (43 year old clergyman)

A few take up the orthodox Catholic position of denying the spiritual and legal possibility of divorce in any circumstance:

> *"Divorce is not so much wrong as strictly speaking impossible – whatever legal fictions we allow. What God has joined together, only God can put asunder, and he does so only by death. The idea that divorce is easy and possible, prevents many from making the effort and practising the self denial which could have made the marriage a success."* (36 year old clergyman)

Equally few of these Church of England clergymen go to the opposite extreme of recommending extension of the existing legal grounds for divorce:

> *"I should support divorce by consent – but it might cause more unhappiness on the whole."* (63 year old clergyman)

Differences of attitude between church-goer and non church-goer suggest that contact with the church has a pronounced influence on attitude to divorce. One in three of the weekly or fortnightly church-goers disapprove of divorce, compared with one in four of those who do not go to Church at all. It is not surprising, therefore, that clergymen as a group show an outlook quite different to that of each of the non-clerical groups – doctors, teachers, street-sample and National Panel; in each of these there are varying elements of what seems to be religiously derived feeling; but also in each of these lay groups the majority approve of divorce according to a practical rather than religious criterion. For just over half the street sample divorce is a necessary evil, to be avoided wherever possible, but better than unhappiness; the religious obstacle of indissoluble and sacred matrimonial views seldom comes explicitly into their views. A 90 year old ex-teacher, for instance, sums up the conflict between religious and lay opinion when he says:

> *"I quite agree with divorce. One comes across the idea that marriages are made in heaven. Rubbish! Often they are made in hell, and should be terminated."*

Churchgoers represent one pocket of resistance to divorce, and another source of opposition is the country. To some extent people think favourable of divorce according to the size of town they live in. Londoners are most favourable of all. But even more marked than this effect of town or country background, is the influence of class or income. The more people earn, the less likely they are to disapprove of divorce:

48% of those earning less than £3 (note 1) a week disapprove of divorce
34% of those earning less than £4 a week   "   "   "   "
35% of those earning between £4 and £5.10 a week disapprove of divorce
26% of those earning between £5.10 and £10   "   "   "
20% of those earning £10 a week disapprove   "   "   "

The income factor, partly a matter of education, is consistent with the general relation between earning capacity and 'free' views on sexual matters. It has already emerged in discussion of sex education and birth control. But in the case of divorce, differences of approval rates are particularly pronounced, and one reason for this may possibly be the relative inaccessibility of divorce to the less well-off. This money aspect of divorce does not often come explicitly into attitudes (only 2% say that divorce should be made easier, and these are not always referring to expense). This is quite clearly not an issue about which many people feel very strongly; but it seems likely that only the better off regard divorce as any sort of practical possibility for themselves, and for people in the lower income groups divorce can safely remain anathema whilst it is out of their personal reach.

Men and women are alike in the extent to which they accept divorce, and age seems to have no influence on attitude. Similarly, there seems to be no relation between attitudes to divorce and marital status, length of engagement prior to marriage, or marriage with or without children. In fact the whole picture seems more or less static, except for the two strong cross-currents of income and religion. The religious influence, however, is by no means only a matter of churchgoing. Much more important than merely whether or not people go to church – more important even than income – is the effect of the type of church people go to. Roman Catholics are more consistently hostile to divorce than any other group we were able to investigate. Opposed to divorce were:

69% of all Roman Catholic church-goers
29% of all Church of England   "   "
29% of all Non-conformist   "   "
27% of all Church of Scotland   "   "

Some Catholics, on the other hand, approve of divorce without apparently considering that they are repudiating their religious teachings; but Catholic conflict on the question of divorce seems less frequent and less severe than the conflict produced by the problem of birth control, with its more immediate personal application:

> "*It's a way out for people who can't stand each other*" (27 year old labourer, Westminster, R.C.)

Only 4% of the Catholic group (consisting of all churchgoers however occasionally) are unreservedly in favour of divorce; whilst an additional 18% agree to it for special cases. But to Catholics 'special cases' is a narrower category than usual, with the emphasis largely on the more legally orthodox exceptions such as adultery and insanity. Even so, it is clear that the Papal denial of divorce under any circumstance does not by any means find inevitable acceptance amongst the members of the Catholic church.

But even amongst non-Catholics and in the group which more or less accepts the principle of divorce, [few] show signs of conflict. There is seldom any enthusiasm about approval, and again and again recurs the proviso that divorce should not be too easy. The practical and humanitarian desire to avoid matrimonial unhappiness by making unhappy husbands and wives free of one another, comes into constant conflict with the fear that divorce may become too frequent. Only one in every fifty says that divorce should be easier; but extension of present divorce grounds would probably be uneasily acceptable to the majority:

> "*That is rather a difficult question. I don't see the point of people living together if they are just rowing and quarrelling all the time. If they are totally unsuited to one another I think they should be divorced, but it should not be made too easy.*" (46 year old housewife (880))

It is difficult to judge precisely what people mean by 'not too easy'. Their reluctance seems stronger than a mere desire to avoid a Hollywood like succession of divorces, and it is rather a stipulation that no divorce should be granted except for serious disagreement between husband and wife. It is here that the hereditary connection between Church opposition to divorce and lay approval of it is at its most obvious – there is still an unquestioned acceptance of the desirability of unbroken, lifelong marriages, even amongst those who may otherwise approve of divorce; second marriages are second best. The emphasis is usually on divorce as a regrettable necessity, to be avoided where ever possible, but not at the expense of happiness:

> "*For a few I know, a divorce would be an advantage. Take my sister, anything would be better than the hell she has to put up with from her husband. But she won't divorce and so she has to go on living like it.*" (34 year old shop assistant, wife of tie-salesman) (533)

> "*Well I think divorce when there can't be any reconciliation, yes, but they should try, especially if there are children. I know, I speak from experience. I had a terrible time with my husband once, and if I could have divorced him then I would. But now we are as happy as ever –*

think divorce should be avoided wherever possible". (42 year old wife of an electrical engineer (663))

Only a minority go further towards a more positive view of divorce:

"I think the best thing to do is to divorce – it cuts out a whole lot of misery and brings happiness." (55 year old widow, Chester)

Even fewer, about one in every fifty, say that divorce should be easier to obtain, especially for poorer people who at present may be unable to afford it:

"It's a good thing. It ought to be made easier still. I know plenty who have no happiness at all, who would be happier with some other partner." (48 year old miner 432)

"If you have got the wrong partner, there should be a law to get a divorce free, not have to spend all that money on it. (35 year old baker's assistant, miner's wife)

One of the most striking results emerging from our material is the gap between legal and popular opinion on the subject of grounds for divorce. Legally, divorce can be granted only for special cases such as adultery, desertion, insanity and cruelty. Disagreement and marital incompatibility are not recognised at all, and where it can be shown that both parties agree in wanting the divorce, it should not legally be granted. Yet every three of our street sample spontaneously and specifically insist that divorce is all right if husband and wife do not get on together; this is the only grounds for divorce that is mentioned by more than a small proportion; adultery occurs very seldom:

"If they're not happy it's no use living together, life is too short. You don't know when you marry what they are like." (45 year old wife of seedsman's assistant)

One in every three of the street sample is opposed to divorce – and it is in the views of this opposition group that the relation between Church and lay opinion again becomes particularly clear. Disapproval of divorce is almost always based on the implied assumption that marriage must be a permanency; sometimes this is more than implied, an explicitly religious objection. Catholics, as in the case of birth control, tend to mention their religion as sole reason for their opposition:

"Being a Catholic I don't agree with it" (29 year old Canteen worker, Westminster)

Opposition to divorce purely as a Church member comes largely from Catholics. But – and here attitudes to divorce differ from attitudes to birth control – it is by no means only Catholics who object to divorce on more broadly religious grounds.

> *"There would never be any divorces if I had my way. They go to Church and swear 'till death do us part', and therefore they should stick it out to the end."* (51 year old Railway Guard, Manchester)

> *"If I was married, I could not be divorced – not in the eyes of God, whatever they said. It's against my religion."* (18 year old discharged soldier, Worcester)

But more frequent than the explicitly religious objection is the assumption that a marriage should last for always. A Greenock O.A.P. for example insists:

> *"Divorce shouldn't be. When you're mated that's for your natural life."*

And another OAP, this time from [....] (341), blames broken 'vows' on to over-hasty marriages:

> *"Once married is married, I say. People should look before they leap and then keep their vows."*

The Christian ethic of lifelong monogamy is very much part of the British conscience. Even though religious reasons are probably seldom ever thought of as grounds for objecting to divorce, there is an imperative flavour of 'should' and 'ought' about replies that suggest morality is the main criterion:

> *"Well, there shouldn't be divorce, If you have happiness in your first husband, you have given all that you have to give."* (66 year old widow, Baptist) (631)

> *"I don't think people should get divorced. They should try and get on the best they can."* (50 year old cleaner porter's wife, Christian Scientist, Westminster)

Perhaps there is also something of the Christian belief in the value of suffering in the replies of those who object to divorce vaguely on the grounds that people should 'put up with' their difficulties:

> *"... No, that's not right. If you make your bed you should lie on it."* (49 year old porter's wife, Pimlico, Church of E.)

Not so very different to the logic that divorce is wrong because people should

> *"I think that many people marry without a full sense of responsibility, thinking that divorce can solve problems if they arise ...."* (27 year old schoolmistress)

Practical reasons for objecting to divorce are much less frequent than ethical ones of principle. One of these is the fear of hurting the children by separating their parents – although a few take the opposite point of view that from the children's angle bickering parents are worse than none. A Rochdale widow is uncertain which is the best answer:

> *"Divorce is a very sad thing when there's little children. Very sad. I've seen some very sad cases. But some people – they're better apart."* (47 year old widow, dentist's receptionist)

Perhaps it is inevitable that, regarding divorce as wrong in itself, people should expect to find unhappiness resulting from it. The trend – of which there are some small indications – towards regarding divorced parents as a better solution for their children than squabbling parents, may be one step away from this way of thinking. This retired Staffordshire miner has a view of divorce that is again possibly a type of wishful thinking:

> *"When you come to divorce there's never no happiness. People should stick together and make the best of their bargain. Nobody asked them to get wed."*

Religious influences on attitudes to divorce are stronger than any other; but where their impact is weakened it seems to be partly a result of conflict with class and income factors. Amongst our National Panel, for instance, although divorce is for the most part conceived in the same terms as amongst the street sample, the morality of monogamy for its own sake is less clearly apparent. Fewer people reject divorce out of hand, and, in particular, fewer reject it purely because they think marriage ought to be for life. Even so, in the group as a whole, there is still the same majority assumption that divorce is an undesirable substitute for lifelong marriages, even though this assumption is less emphatic and tends to have a less moralistic tone:

> *"A divorce is better in every way, in my opinion, than a loveless home. If one has make a mistake, it is better to be able to remedy it."*
> (38 year old woman secretary, panel member – herself divorced)

Again there is the same insistence on incompatibility as a ground for divorce, again tempered by fear of divorce becoming 'too easy'. This 49 year old Yorkshire housewife, for instance, goes much further than most [....]. She represents the vanguard of pro-divorce opinion:

> *"Divorce should be made as easy as marriage. If two people don't get on there is no sense in their living together, hating each other. It's hard luck on the children, but surely better for them to live with one parent than with two who loathe each other. Marriage should be a civil contract. The church should be abolished!"*

The role of children in divorce is more frequently present in the minds of this more educated group than of the street sample. Of this group one in nine qualifies his approval of divorce with plans for the children; on the other hand there are many others – considerably more than amongst the street sample – who believe that children are better off away from unhappy parents. A middle aged housewife reasons:

> *"I can't see that it helps children to be brought up in a house where hatred or even indifference reigns!"*

Doctors and teachers show much the same pattern of opinion about divorce as that of our National Panel, but probably because they are more religiously inclined! Approval is slightly less frequent amongst them than in the Panel group, although still much more frequent than in the street sample; but again the emphasis is a two-sided one, equally pointing to the need for avoiding divorce wherever possible – and to granting it where it is really necessary:

> *"When a marriage has failed from any cause after a genuine attempt to make it a success then with-holding a divorce is unnecessary cruelty."* (39 year old doctor)

> *"It is probably necessary in certain cases, notably those of insanity and total desertion, but I think it is granted far too freely."* (29 year old doctor)

> *"I am wholly in favour of divorce, provided safeguards against abuse are efficient."* (54 year old schoolmaster)

But explicitly religious opposition to divorce is inclined to slip into the views of these doctors and teachers, in a way that occurs to a considerably lesser extent amongst the Panel – and more even than amongst the street sample, for whom disapproval of divorce is more usually based on vaguely moral reasonings. A middle aged schoolteacher, for instance, a member of the Church of England, feels very strongly that divorce is religiously impossible:

> *"As marriage should be the union of two soul-mates by the Almighty, only He can nullify the same, and the present system of divorce is a farce; and as in my opinion Man cannot make a marriage, neither can he make a divorce. The present legal procedure is solely a means of*

*putting shekels into the pockets of certain members of the legal pro-
fession!"*

More typical, but still unrepresentative – this time in its enthusiasm – is the
view of this 50 year old schoolmaster, of no particular religious beliefs:

*"Divorce is the most sensible thing to do when a marriage has failed.
What about the children? Very difficult, but it is better for them to live
with one parent than in an unhappy home with two."*

Generally, most people accept the principle of divorce reluctantly, uneasy lest
it becomes too frequent a practice, but at the same time firmly preferring broken marriages to unhappy ones. It is significant that those experiencing an
unsatisfactory parental marriage are slightly more in favour of divorce than
those whose background has left them ignorant of such circumstances.
Particularly, the better off people are financially, and the less their religious
inclinations, the more likely they are to look with favour on divorce; even
more marked, the further their views diverge from the Catholic Church, the
more they are inclined to accept the principle of second marriage, even after
the first has been broken by nothing more dramatic than unhappiness. It
seems likely that many people are unaware that this principle of divorce on
grounds of simple incompatibility, which so many of them recommend, is not
recognised by the law; if they did realise this their feelings might be stronger.
Possibly if religious beliefs continue to decline, and if divorce becomes easier as well as cheaper, and therefore readily accessible to more than the middle class, it will become even more widely accepted than it is at present.
Except amongst the standard Catholics and church goers, opposition to
divorce is less bitter and less emotional than opposition to almost any of the
other subject [s] of the investigation.

Notes

1 In the case of housewives or dependants, the income is that of the family's chief
   wage earner. In any case it is exclusive of bonus earnings.

Part D, Outside Marriage

Chapter Seven: Sex Outside Marriage

Reluctance to surrender wholesale the principle of life-long monogamy makes the 'man in the street' uneasy about divorce; to an even greater extent it leads him to condemn sex relations outside marriage. More people are more strongly opposed to extra-marital relations than they are to any of the other subjects of this survey. The only groups providing an exception to this rule are doctors, clergymen and Mass-Observation's National Panel – the first two slightly, the latter very much inclined, to prefer extra-marital relations to prostitution. In each group, the numbers disapproving of extra-marital relations were:

24% of the National Panel
63% of the street sample
65% of doctors
75% of teachers
90% of clergymen

This is the usual pattern, with the National Panel taking up what seems to be the vanguard of changing opinion, clergymen were to the rear, and the street sample effecting a compromise between the two outlooks. But in this case of sex relations outside marriage, doctors and teachers are more, rather than – as in other cases – less disapproving than the street sample, probably because convention itself has strong feelings about extra-marital relations affecting the replies of these professional groups, who are inclined to be influenced by what they feel to be socially proper. In any case, there is a clear picture of Church and conventional opposition to extra-marital sex relations, an opposition which is to some extent worn down by the counter influences of class and educational level, working alongside with religious apathy. Within the street sample group differences reflect these influences. Opposed to extra-marital relations are:

73% of all weekly church goers
54% of all non-church goers

64% of people leaving school up to and including 15 years
50% of all leaving school after $16\frac{1}{2}$
68% of all living in rural areas
50% of all Londoners
67% of all women
57% of all men
64% of all married people over 30
48% of all single people over 30

Income and class differences show the same pattern as that of education. Age (excluding the marriage factor) and whether or not married people have children makes no apparent difference. Roman Catholic and Non-Conformist church goers are slightly more inclined than members of the Church of England to repudiate extramarital relations, but generally the most pronounced influence is one of strength of religious belief rather than of actual denomination, conflicting with the less clearly pronounced factor of education, and possibly, Leftish political outlook (note 1).

In attitude to sex, education seems to clear the way towards some sanctioning of unmarried sex relations. Investigating sex behaviour, on the other hand, Kinsey in America found the reverse trend. How far this reflects a cleavage between attitude and habit, how far merely a difference between English and American patterns of behaviour, it is difficult to judge. That the latter is the case, however, is suggested by income differences in experience of pre-marital relations within Mass-Observation's National Panel; these differences can give rise only to tentative conclusions, since they are small enough to be possibly merely a reflection of sampling [procedures]; but such as they are, they show a tendency for a lighter incidence of pre-marital experience in the higher income groups. 66% of these earning over £15 a week have experienced sex relations before marriage, compared with 49% of those with a weekly income of less than £10. Looking at all the evidence as a whole, habit and attitude together, it seems at least likely that education accompanies not only a lower code of sexual ethics, but also, in direct contrast to the situation uncovered by Kinsey in America, an additional looseness of actual sexual behaviour.

Results from the Panel group as a whole show that it is not only the marriage sanctioning of sex relations, but also the principle of life-long monogamy, that is loosening. As many as 39% of all the married members of our National Panel have had sex relations before marriage with their husband or wife; and an additional 16%, bringing the total proportion up to more than half, [....] had experienced sexual intercourse with someone, fiancé, or otherwise, before marriage. These figures are consistently rather lower for women than for men – but even so, one wife in every three had intercourse with her husband before marriage, and one in four had pre-marital relations with someone other than her present husband. On the whole it seems true to say that someone who indulged in pre-marital relations at all, is also likely to have intercourse before marriage with their future husband or wife. The 55% who experienced some sort of pre-marriage sex relations are made up of the following sub-groups:

22% (of all married people) have had pre-marital relations both with their present spouse and others
17% have confined their pre-marital relations to their present spouse
16% have had pre-marital relations, but not with their present spouse

In other words, in this group at least, it is a minority only, but a largish minority, that keeps its intended husband or wife in a category separate from pre-marital adventures.

Of the 38% married members of the National Panel who have experienced pre-marital relations with men or women other than their present husband or wife, only a very small minority have confined themselves to a single additional partner; most have had intercourse with 2, 3, or 4 different partners beside their present spouse; 5% have had relations with a number of partners that ranges from 7 to 20 or more. Men appear to have a greater variety of partners than women.

But marriage proves a handicap to sexual variation. Although a third of our married group had experienced pre-marital relations with someone other than their present husband or wife, only 22% have supplemented marital relations since their marriage. Again, men prove rather bolder in this respect than women; one husband in four, compared with one wife in every five, admits to experience of sex relations outside marriage.

These results [are] from a group which is below average in religious belief and ties, and above average in educational level and Leftish politics; unfortunately we have no valid comparative results for the population as a whole. Illegitimacy statistics, however, throw some light on the question – 1939 figures show that in 418 out of every 1,000 marriages where the wife was under 20, she was also pregnant. Taking all age groups together, 30% of all first births were either illegitimate or conceived out of wedlock – despite increasing knowledge of birth control. There is ample evidence for assuming that at least one person in three, probably more, has intercourse either before or outside marriage; although unsanctioned relations may be more frequent amongst the higher educational groups and the religiously apathetic, the man in the street is at least not so far behind as his spoken attitude would suggest.

Investigating the facts of sex behaviour, a clear distinction arises between pre-marital relations between two people who are later to be married and more casual forms of unmarried intercourse. The first appears to be the more common. Investigating sex attitudes, we left it to the people questioned to point out differences between one sort of extra-marital relation and another; and it quickly became clear that the same distinction between casual relations and 'serious' is often a pre-requisite of extra-marital relations generally. Sex relations between two people who are in love, engaged, or somehow unable somehow unable to marry, are far more often condoned than sex relations based largely on physical attraction alone. [A] case history, for instance, collected during the course of the present survey from a [....] girl in a North country industrial town, is typical in the consistency with which it rounds off descriptions of pre-marital incidents with 'I loved him a lot' – even if it is untypical in the frequency with which such incidents occur [.....] (note 2). To this girl feeling is as important a sanction to intercourse as marriage itself; but even so, marriage has not lost its importance. There is a faintly illogical ring to her desire to 'keep something' – in this case, nudity – in reserve for marriage when it does occur.

Questioning doctors, teachers and clergymen, we provided a ready-made distinction between pre-marital and extra-marital relations. The figure quoted earlier for these three groups refers to pre-marital relations only; each group is a little more opposed to sex relations outside marriage by married people. But, just as the street sample occasionally insists on drawing the distinction for itself, generally, amongst these people with a somewhat more rigid sexual ethic, the distinction makes little practical difference. Clergymen in particular object to any sex relations unsanctioned by a marriage tie. Whether the relation is a straightforward unmarried one, or whether it is complicated by third party husbands or wives, seems to them more or less irrelevant; they are almost unanimous in their condemnation of such behaviour. This middle aged clergyman is exceptional:

"In the case of two young people deeply in love it is surely readily forgivable. As a cynical satisfaction of the sexual instinct it is totally wrong. It is a great pity that economic conditions make the postponement of marriage so often necessary. Extra-marital relations are wrong, of course, but for a man whose wife is completely unresponsive, celibacy can be a great strain...."

The more usual practice is to call unmarried sex relations fornication or adultery, and as such condemn them out of hand:

"Pre-marital sexual intercourse is the sin of fornication, and is therefore wrong. Extra-marital sexual intercourse is the sin of adultery and is therefore wrong." (35 year old clergyman)

One middle-aged clergyman felt that extra-marital relations 'should be punishable by law'. Another sees even pre-marital intercourse as a source of disharmony and dissatisfaction:

"If you mean between engaged couples, it is not only 'immoral', but thoroughly injurious. The wife is 'stale' before marriage; while neither can be expected to trust the other, remembering their pre-marital habits."

But the usual course is for clergymen to condemn all unmarried relations simply as a sin. Doctors and teachers, on the other hand, in any case less consistently opposed to extra-marital intercourse, are a little more inclined to see
the matter from a personal point of view. To them, unmarried sex relations
are usually not sinful but immoral – a crime against society rather than God;
and in addition they are just not necessary. The necessity criterion appears
amongst the views of sympathetic and hostile alike:

> *"Reason tells me that pre-marital sexual intercourse concerns only the
> people involved; upbringing and its prejudices makes me condemn it.
> Personal experience inclines me to commend it as a means of acquir-
> ing technique.*
>
> *I dislike the thought of extra-marital relations intensely. But (this
> may be mere male trade unionism) I recognise that for a man of 40 or
> 50, with a wife of similar age, the problem may be rather pressing. As
> I am 16 years older than my wife, perhaps I am somewhat smug."* (40
> year old headmaster)

On the other hand:

> *"Extra marital relations represent moral degeneration. Sexual inter-
> course is not any man's – or woman's – necessity."* (58 year old
> schoolmaster)

> *"Pre-marital sexual intercourse is unnecessary, usually completely
> selfish, and I advise that it should not be indulged in."* (56 year old
> schoolmaster)

Doctors are more inclined to take advantage of the distinction between extra-
and pre-marital relations, discriminating in favour of the latter. Again, biological and social yardsticks are inclined to show through their attitudes:

> *"Premarital sexual intercourse is necessary if everyone has to marry
> in the late twenties. The period of active sexual life is short for a
> woman, and she may well have reached the middle of that period
> before she marries."* (40 year old surgeon)

> *"I am against it. This is promiscuity which courts venereal disease on
> the one hand, and divorce on the other; an anti-social practice."* (47
> year old surgeon)

The moral criterion is still usually the basic one. Even where they are
approved, unmarried sex relations still tend to be regarded as a lesser evil, for
the most part only desirable where present day society or special circumstances – age discrepancies, divergent sexual appetites, the improbability of

marriage, etc. – make them necessary. Relatively few of these doctors and teachers prefer even pre-marital relations for positive rather than negative reasons. [....]. Where they do, it is usually on the grounds that premarital sex relations are sex-educational:

> *"Pre-marital intercourse is essential for a man and probably advisable for the average woman. Physical clumsiness in a man can ruin a marriage, it also helps each to realise that there is more in marriage than mere sexual gratification."* (39 year old doctor)

But generally, where doctor and teachers are more inclined than clergyman to favour unmarried intercourse, it is because they are more inclined to suspect that the current standards of morality are not always easy to carry out. One 37 year old psychiatrist, discussing pre-marital intercourse, says that he is opposed to it, but -

> *"... allowance must be made for the few – say 5 – 10% – of our weaker brethren"*

Most clergymen are unwilling to make allowance for the 'weaker brethren'. The man in the street, on the other hand, puts their percentage at a very much higher figure, and is correspondingly more inclined – even than teachers or doctors – to sympathise with unmarried sex relations. Even so, two-thirds of our street sample disapprove of sex relations between unmarried people. Most of this large unfavourable group replied briefly but in unambiguous terms: *"That's wrong"*, *"I don't agree with that"*, *"It's filthy"*, *"Well I think that's awful"*, *"Oh no, that's not done, that's lust"*. Like doctors and teachers, they object to extra-marital relations, not as a sin but because they regard them as immoral and wrong. The few that elaborate their reasons for objecting, either explaining like one young baker's assistant that *"You can't expect your future wife to be pure and clean"*, or else condemn unmarried sex as lust, or take the third alternative of venturing into humanitarian rather than realistic arguments – broken homes, false happiness, etc. Regulating unorthodox sex relations as lust is generally felt to be sufficient argument against them – again there is the feeling that sex for its own sake must be wrong, just as control for its own sake is probably right; marriage gives dignity to sex:

> *"I don't believe in it, it's not right, it's going like animals."* (70 year old painter and decorator (621))

A taxi cab proprietor objects to any infringement of the conventions:

> *"I feel very strongly about this. I've seen a lot of the harm it causes. I may say my wife and I have dropped one or two people who weren't playing the game, we didn't think they were worth knowing."*

Amongst those who accept extra-marital relations, there is again much of the 'faut mieux' feeling that appeared in the replies of doctors and teachers. Sex relations between unmarried people are seldom welcomed, more often condoned, and almost always there is the defensive attitude of the uneasy minority. Again positive arguments are rare:

> *"You can't stop the feeling. I agree with it. It's to try people out – you never want to buy a pig in a poke..."* (37 year old steeple jack, (622))

And a young (231) park-keeper:

> *"The female body is really made for that sort of thing".*

There is occasional evidence of a belief that unmarried couples living 'in sin' are happier than married couples. A middle aged housewife, for instance:

> *"Some times they are much happier than if they were married, there's some cases even in this town I know of".*

Less enthusiastic, but still placing the emphasis on positive rather than purely substitutive values, is approval of extra-marital relations as quite simply 'natural'. And this middle-aged steelworker even goes to the Bible for justification:

> *"That's really mutual consent, isn't it, and in the Bible if you read it closely, it says that even if one is married and the other is not, if there is mutual consent it isn't committing adultery."*

[....]

> *"That's nature. You can't beat nature, can you. If you get to that, well it's just natural, I suppose."* (65 year old building labourer (621))

And a young labourer: (531)

> *"It's nature taking its course, if you ask us"*

But much more usually, extra-marital relations are conceded rather than granted whole-heartedly. There are special circumstances when they may be justified – inability to marry for one reason or another, the strain of engagement, separation between husband and wife. Again there is the frequent distinction between couples intending marriage, and more casual, temporary, affairs. And equally important with the special circumstances argument is the concession to biology; men are human after all.

A (722) ship builder, Roman Catholic concedes:

"The Church says it's a sin, but I can see that sometimes a couple can't help themselves."

An old age pensioner says, sympathetically, *"You can't help it sometimes"*. And a dock labourer refers the matter back to his own impulse:

"It's hard to say. As far as I can see everybody does it. If I was single I wouldn't refuse, would I."

About one percent of the whole street sample refuse to judge something which they admit they themselves have done. Considerably more frequent is a suggestion of probable personal experience – often accompanied by a feeling of guilt or defensiveness; they are inclined to say that 'there is nothing against it' – rather than what there is for unmarried sex relations. And this lorry driver, for instance, is quite candid about the divergence between what he does, and what he feels he ought to do:

"That shouldn't be allowed. Just because I do it, I don't think it's right."

Occasional men, thinking along contrary lines to the more usual exoneration of engaged couples, say they would have pre-marital relations only with a girl they did not intend to marry. Sometimes a girl's refusal of sex relations is even regarded as a pre-requisite to accepting her as a wife; but this seems to be largely a working class attitude, and even then exceptional:

"If I'm going around just for a good time I don't mind taking a girl, but if I was going with a girl I was wanting to marry I wouldn't touch her" (23 year old builder's labourer, 742)

And a 20 year old Londoner described to an observer how he had had intercourse with ten different girls (including a prostitute) but has not had intercourse with his fiancée:

"After I had been going with her for two months, I tried to go all the way with her, but it wouldn't work. She wants a white wedding and marriage in a Church, and to be a virgin. I agree with her and I don't try any more. When I first tried and she refused I thought she was the right girl. If she had gone with me I don't think I would gave gone out long with her because she would just have been another girl."

One in fourteen metaphorically shrug their shoulders and say that it is up to the individual to decide whether or not they should go in for unmarried sex relations. Of the whole sample, analysis revealed the following attitude proportions. Out of every 100 questioned:

63   disapproved of sex relations between unmarried people
1   disapproved if children were involved
8   approved of, or were not against it
7   said it was a matter for the individuals concerned
5   were in favour under some circumstances
5   were in favour provided it was a 'serious' relationship, or between engaged couples
1   was in favour provided no third party was involved
1   said he had done it himself
5   were undecided
4   had mixed feelings
1   refused to answer
1   gave miscellaneous replies
(a few gave replies belonging to more than one category)

Even though one third of this national cross-section did not actually disapprove of extra-marital relations, only one in seven gave even lukewarm unqualified approval. There is certainly no easy or wide-spread acceptance of sex relations outside marriage in the population as a whole. However, there is some evidence for assuming that it is the higher educational groups who tend to provide a model for changing attitudes, and it is the more educated who are most inclined to accept unmarried intercourse. This is particularly apparent amongst workers of Mass-Observation's National Panel who, as a group, show a majority at least partially in favour of sex relations between unmarried people. Out of every 100 Panel members:

     (24 were against extra-marital relations
29   (3 disapproved if children were involved
     (2 said they would not do it themselves
15   were in favour of, or not against extra-marital relations
18   were in favour of them under some circumstances
18   were in favour, provided it was a 'serious' relationship or between engaged couples
15   said it was a matter for the individuals concerned
5   were in favour provided no third party was involved
1   said he would do it himself
8   had mixed feelings
3   gave miscellaneous replies

Although 'ifs' and 'buts' and special circumstances abound, there is in this group much less reluctance to admit the principle of extra-marital relations. Moral criteria are less frequently referred to than amongst the street sample, giving place instead to humanitarian considerations of expediency and individual satisfaction. More or less typical in general attitude, for instance, is this elderly Panel member:

"So long as each party is sure that he or she knows what they are about, and there is no feeling of 'guilt', I see nothing against extra-marital relations and much for it".

A draughtsman:

"I've no objection, providing one doesn't eventually flit from one person to another."

And a commercial traveller:

"It's O.K. if the people concerned are content. Half the taboos always came from the possible child. Birth control has altered this and much else."

There are still restrictions on approval, but they have changed their form. Provided no one else is harmed, and provided the individuals accept the responsibility for their actions, little else is relevant:

"It's a matter of personal morality. It doesn't really matter what they do as long as they behave in a responsible way." (55 year old museum director)

Sometimes there is not even any reference to provisos *"Ha, free love!"* says one young man, *"Live and let live."* The emphasis in this group is on the individual – on personal morality, individual responsibility, [....] and the impossibility of any absolute standards of morality. Secure in the knowledge of their educational background, this group is prepared not merely tentatively to take up a different attitude to the conventional one, but even to take the offensive, suggesting that convention and morality themselves may be in need of change:

"Extra-marital relations are quite in order. It all depends on the physical and psychological needs of the persons concerned. The present moral code makes for too little allowance for individual variation." (37 year old man, engaged in agricultural research)

Where members of the Panel group are against extra-marital relations, it is again to some extent in individual terms rather than in terms of absolute morality that they repudiate it – although moralistic disapproval is by no means infrequent. But at least equally often they reject unmarried sex relations because they feel that this is in practice not likely to lead to happiness:

"I am against sex relations between unmarried people, because I feel it would spoil something that would otherwise be an experience confined to two people only." (40 year old housewife)

"In actual practice it doesn't work out so well; quite frequently the woman has to pay, and the mental effect on the two sexes is quite different." (43 year old housewife)

If it is true that present day higher educational attitudes are travelling down the social scale, if the drift away from the Church continues, together with the shift of emphasis from absolute Church derived morality to morality based on social and humanitarian sanctions, then the Panel group are expressing something of the general attitudes of tomorrow. If that is the case, acceptance of extra-martial relations would become less reluctant, and a majority rather than a minority attitude.

Notes

1   A process of holding [constant] first the education, then the income, factor, and breaking results down by the other, suggested that, as far as it is possible to separate the two, education is a more decisive factor than income. Unfortunately our survey left this factor uninvestigated; but to some extent its effect can be gauged by the difference of outlook between the M-O National Panel, an abnormally Leftish group, and the street sample or teacher or doctor groups.

[2   This case history was in the first draft of the *Sunday Pictorial* articles and was to have been included in the chapter at this point. However, through editing processes it was removed from the published article and no longer exists in a discernible form in the archive materials.]

CHAPTER Eight: Prostitution

"Proverbs, chapter 7, is the Divine answer. 'The prostitute's love is the way to hell, going down to the chambers of death'."

This elderly vicar takes an extreme view of prostitution, but one which is not entirely divorced from popular opinion. The mention of prostitution aroused more indignation and disgust amongst the people we interviewed than any other single aspect of sex; even sexual abnormality tend to be discussed with more toleration, if perhaps also with more simple disgust and physical lack of comprehension. But it seems likely that some of at least of the repressive moralistic disapproval with which prostitution is regarded is itself based on a misapprehension; Sunday newspaper publicity given to the subject perhaps leads to exaggerated ideas of its extent. Certainly our survey suggests that prostitution, in its usual sense, plays a slighter part in our national life than is often imagined; although there is no doubt that 'black spots' exist, they have to be looked for.

Naturally, however, assessment of the extensiveness of prostitution must inevitably remain dependent on the outlook of the person reading the facts. For instance, one in four of the male members of Mass-Observation's National Panel admitted experience of sex relations with prostitutes. Since their experience was in most of these cases at least five years distant, some people would take this as indicating a relatively low overall incidence. To others, on the other hand, experience of prostitution for one man in four must appear a startlingly high figure. With the possibility of such varying interpretations in mind, the facts, in so far as we were able to discover them, must be left to speak for themselves and [....] to clarify the factual situation before going on to discuss the attitudes to which the facts give rise.

The prostitution picture in our two main study areas, Churchtown and Steeltown, provided an interesting contrast. In the former, the Chief Constable told an Investigator: -

"There are no known prostitutes operating at all. There may be a few enthusiastic amateurs, but they conduct themselves quietly and

privately, so I cannot say anything about them. I don't think they are a problem – there are no black spots. We would give them short shrift if there were any; soliciting may be practised in a limited way in the public houses – but it is doubtful. We would know about it if it was going on."

Interviews with other town officials, as well as informal conversation and observation, more or less confirmed this story. According to the town's Assistant Medical Officer, prostitution in Churchtown is not even the main source of the town's V.D.:-

"The worst spot is around the bottom of B..... St. There are one or two pubs there which are the source of most of the V.D. in Churchtown. I've asked men time and time again where they met the woman, and they say in one of those pubs. There must be a small hard core of carriers in those pubs. No, they are not paid prostitutes. The men always tell me that they didn't pay for it...."

In so far as prostitution exists in Churchtown, it seems to be prostitution of a very subdued kind. And even in Steeltown, the Chief Probation Officer felt himself able to say:

"There's nothing at all outstanding here as regards sexual morality. The prostitute problem is very small, confined to a few round the docks – but it's not a serious problem. It only affects a few ... There are no more than two dozen prostitutes in the town, and these are known to and recognised by the Police. In addition there are those who go on board the ships; most of these are under twenty years old – there's no demand for the older ones on the ships. What they do is get the Gazette and see what ships are coming in, and according to the ship they know which pub to go to. They like to keep to their regular ships, although they're not entirely averse to a change."

As we pointed out before, however, what constitutes a problem depends entirely on the angle from which the matter is approached. From the Church point of view, the picture in Steeltown is not so encouraging. A Church of England parson, for instance, told an Investigator:-

"There is a lot of immorality in town, and I would say that Steeltown is fairly representative of an industrial town. You must remember that this is a port – and as such, sailors are coming; where there's a port there is almost inevitably a fairly flourishing 'Red Light' business – it's straight commercial prostitution. The girls are taken to the boats, and the foreign sailors give them money, cigarettes, and that."

And the physician in charge of the Steeltown V.D. Clinic is almost equally gloomy:-

> *"Steeltown is a port, you know. The V.D. figures are very heavy. We have 200 a month of new cases – they have been exposed to possible infection. Incidence of syphilis has not gone down; a lot of Scandinavian seamen come here – they're a pretty tough crowd; they bring it to the town. The Francis Drake is a prostitutes haunt – all round that area – in the pubs and that. Steeltown blokes drift down that way as well, but essentially they cater for the seamen...."*

Generally it is clear from these official interviews that prostitution in Steeltown, in so far as it forces itself upon people's attention, is mainly confined only to the dock area, with an additional sprinkling around the stations. Naturally, town officials may be over-willing to give a good report of their town; but on the whole observation by a skilled Investigator supported their views. Following up the unanimous suggestion that the dock area was a 'black spot', however, observations were made in some of the most notorious pubs. Reports indicated that pick-ups for prostitution purposes here were completely frank and undisguised. Here are a few extracts from one report made in the Francis Drake:

> *"The Investigator entered the Francis Drake public house (on the edge of the dock area) at 8.30 pm. and left at 10.10 pm.*
>
> *A 50 year old big buxom tart, hard, wan face, heavily made up, satin blouse, and blue costume, seen all her best days, is talking to them all. Then she stands up with a half pint glass two-thirds full of bitter balanced on her head. She keeps her body absolutely still from the waist upwards, but moves and sways her lower abdomen and hips in a most voluptuous and fascinating manner. Men's eyes cannot but help to be attracted to that suggestively rolling mass of flesh. The Indians all had their eyes fixed on her body as she swayed it. She stopped after about a minute, laughed something about 'keeping it down', and sat down.*
>
> *Ten minutes later a 45 year-old labouring man from the town comes into the room, looks around, sees this woman sitting opposite and calls her "'ere, 'ere" and beckons her with curling finger. She smiles and says 'No, not tonight. I'm sorry, I'm on ice'. The labouring man grimaces and walks out of the door.*
>
> *A Swedish sailor and a girl sit each on a stool facing each other. He moves his hand up and down her thigh, she looks at him and smiles – they are talking on and off during the whole time. She opens her legs wide as she sits on the stool, and her short skirt exposes above her knees as she does so. He looks at her legs thus revealed. She again*

> *smiles and opens and closes her legs slowly. He holds her and whispers into her ear – she smiles in response. ....*
>
> *A Swedish seaman comes into the room – he has two black eyes. A 20 year old girl catches him by the hand sand sings "Two lovely Black Eyes" to him. He says 'You come with me?' 'No Bluey', she replies, 'I can't go with you.' He 'I want you', She – 'Yes well, I don't want you'. He sits beside her for a while, arm round her waist, talking. She laughs at him and eventually pushes him away....*
>
> *About three tall, good looking, well dressed Swedish seamen come into the room. Each has a young prostitute on his arm, probably picked up in other pubs or in the streets. The three pairs sit down. The men drink beer, the women double gins. They sit close together, the three men with their arms round the girls' waists or shoulders. During the singing in accompaniment to the accordion, these three pairs sing, faces close together, swaying their bodies in time with the music. The women are far more affected by their drinks than the men. After about forty-five minutes or so these three pairs leave, the girls hanging on to the arms of the men – the men seem to be hurrying them out of the pub ....*
>
> *The rest of the female clientele apparently consists of almost entirely professional prostitutes, there for the object of gaining their contact, usually a foreign seaman, occasionally a Steeltown man. The bulk of the male clientele would seem to consist of foreign seamen there for the purpose of getting drunk and picking up a prostitute."*

That is prostitution at its most open, but it must be remembered that this account describes events in only one relatively small area of a large dock-side town in which the Probation Officer, summing up his opinion of the total position, is able to say that he does not regard prostitution as a serious problem. The picture, moreover, does not seem to be very different even in London. 'Pockets of vice' are much less frequently encountered than is often imagined; a social investigator who had spent a number of years working as a spare-time prostitute in Soho, had never come across either pornographic films or organised brothels – although other evidence shows that she was wrong in believing that organised brothels, at least, do not exist in London (note 1). Here are extracts from a report on one, collected by a woman journalist who spent three months living in the house:

> *"The brothel is run by May, the procuress, fiftyish, who no longer works as a prostitute except to take on the abnormal cases. She has three women working for her. Bet, from the slums of Liverpool, about 30 years, brought up in squalor, left home to take a dull job in London, and, bored, took to prostitution for the glamour of the money. She is good at her job and proud of it. Mary, fiftyish, was married to an Indian Army man. The marriage went on the rocks, and she*

and she returned to England and drink, pubs and parties, finally drifting into prostitution. More cultured than most, she is a bit above everyone else and is regarded as such. She takes the more refined clients – a schoolmaster and a male nurse for instance. Chris, about 24, happily married to a house painter, has three children. Began prostitution by frequenting Central London dance halls, getting drunk, and finally invited into prostitution by May. Husband object-ed at first, then got to like having the extra money .... Chris, Mary and Bet each live on the outskirts of London and come to work every day; they pay May £1 out of the money for every client, and keep what is over – usually at least 10/- ... May has a regular clientele, members of which ring her up on average about four or five times a year; amongst them is a theatre agent, a printer, a sailor, a crippled musician, and a commercial traveller. Most are over 30, mostly a suburban married type periodically out for a good time. May keeps up her clientele list by watching the Soho pubs, making contacts there. In bad financial patches the girls themselves go out to the pubs or the streets for pick-ups. Men are allowed 20 minutes at the most, preliminaries are avoid-ed because they waste time. Because of her care in accepting clients, and because of rigorous washing regulations and using of special sheaths, cases of VD are so far unknown here. So far there has also been a similar immunity from arrest ...."

Unorganised prostitutes, working independently, are of course plentiful in London, particularly in and around Piccadilly; but away from central London, especially away from certain pockets of central London, there is rel-atively little open evidence of them. One exception to this is a street in a London suburb, notorious for the prostitutes who live there:

"The prostitutes live in the houses on one side, the other side is rela-tively free of them. The women sit in their windows, and the men walk up and down the street outside; a prostitute makes a sign to a man, and he comes in for twenty minutes or so. She charges about 10/- a time, and has three or four men in a day. The men tend to be a 'dodgy' looking type – they look as if they might live alone in furnished rooms, not the sort with a wife and family."

This for London is a very exceptional set-up – and once again represents just one little centre of prostitution in a large area relatively free of it. The pene-trative and observational side of this plotting survey was of necessity sketchy; but so far as it went, it suggested very strongly that professional prostitution at least is of relatively minor importance in the life of our towns and cities as a whole.

Our observational material was necessarily confined to prostitution as a full-time job. Amateur prostitution may be much more common; but this shades off into extra-marital relations and the precise line of division between them is often hard to discover. How frequent, for instance, is amateur prostitution of this type – and is it prostitution or is it merely a matter of extra-marital relations?

> *"Gwendoline, friend of a friend of mine, came to our flat the other day and asked if she might borrow our spare room the following night to sleep with a West Indian boy-friend. We agreed, reluctantly. The next night she came with the boy friend. He brought us presents – food and cigarettes, etc. and he brought presents for her too. Then they went to bed. My friend says she has a lot of these Colonial boy friends, and sleeps with most of them on different nights, always in return for presents. But she also has a respectable and quite profitable office job. Is she a prostitute? Did our flat turn into a sort of brothel when we accepted presents for the loan of our room?"*

Whether or not this is a case of prostitution equally with the more clear cut cases quoted earlier is not for us to say. Only when a more comprehensive survey is able to follow on this preliminary one will it be more possible to put all the behaviour ingredients of prostitution and extra-marital relations into proportion in the picture as a whole.

This is the behaviour set-up of prostitution; in its context the more comprehensive picture of attitudes that follows can be integrated into its setting. Disapproval is not only strong but general; alone amongst all the subjects we discussed with people in this investigation, prostitution has a majority against it in every group separately surveyed. Even Mass-Observation's National Panel, much more favourably disposed towards extra-marital relations than any of our other samples, has a 51% majority against prostitution and three out of every 5 of the general population expresses disapproval.

In terms of simple approval and disapproval measurement, the only really striking difference of opinion reflects a cleavage between the clerical and lay outlook. This difference, however, is even clearer when comments are subjected to detailed content analysis. Although both groups, Church and non-clerical alike, look at the matter chiefly in individual terms, clergymen tend most of all to stress the non-moral humanitarian angle whilst lay people more often both pity and blame the prostitute. And secondly, whilst the clergyman's concern with the individual leads him to condemn prostitution as an institution out of hand, the same approach is more inclined to lead particularly the more educated of the non-clerical groups to consider the problem in its social setting of origin and cure. In contrast with the vicar quoted at the beginning of this chapter, for instance, a 26 year old surveyor considers that prostitution:

> *"would disappear under a better-run society – with earlier marriage, easier divorce, less prudery. Until then it is a necessary evil. No supply without the demand."*

And a 34 year old hairdresser takes an even more matter-of-fact view:

"I've no interest in the matter. There is the demand and therefore the supply. Many of these women think it is easy money. I feel sorry for those who practice it."

But it is largely the professional Churchman, speaking in his professional capacity, who stands apart from other groups. Perhaps because the official Church attitude to prostitution is less often brought to the notice of the ordinary man than its views on, for instance, divorce, extra-marital relations and birth control, the churchgoer lags behind his leaders and, to some extent at least, makes up his own mind. But even so church-goers are more inclined to condemn prostitution than members of any other social group; and once again education provides the biggest counter influence, probably because it tends to shift the terms of reference from exclusively moral to at least partially biological and social. The question changes from 'is prostitution right?' to 'is prostitution necessary?'.

But at a verbal level at least, prostitution is the subject of deep and widespread disapproval and disgust. Most unfavourable replies take the form either of simple disgust or moral indignation, expressions like 'disgusting', 'terrible', or 'shocking' occurring about equally with the more matter of fact statement 'I don't agree with that'. Roughly every second person shows one or other of these or similar reactions, whilst an additional 14% say more forcibly that prostitution should be stamped out. Once again those who condemn represent the firmly entrenched majority, whilst the minority who condone prostitution elaborate their comments more defensively. Perhaps because of this majority complacency, practical suggestions as to ways and means of forcibly eradicating prostitution are – except amongst the more socially-concerned middle classes – relatively infrequent. The usual reaction is the verbal equivalent of a disapproving sigh.

But it is interesting that even in disapprobation there is often this underlying suggestion of acceptance that is implied by resignation; for the most part it is only where moral indignation is replaced by consideration of the problem in social terms that this sense of futility entirely disappears. The contrast between the two approaches can be seen in the two following quotations, the first from a socially-minded middle-aged clergyman – not entirely untypical of his kind, the second from a young Shrewsbury lorry-driver:

"One cannot too strongly condemn prostitution, but it has been partly due to social conditions which must be changed. The prostitute should be helped spiritually, medically and psychologically."

"I don't believe in that. Every prostitute should be deported and put on an island of their own."

This young lorry-driver's opinion is not a great deal more vehement than the average view, but the suggestion of futility even in the very extravagance of his solution is fairly clear. There is often a feeling of temporariness about attitudes to prostitution, signs that once the interviewer has disappeared round the corner the matter will be dismissed from mind; reactions to extra-marital relations generally seem much sturdier and more lasting, and contain more indications of realistic, active opposition. It may be that prostitution is to some extent felt to exist relatively water-tight from society as a whole – whilst much rejection of unmarried intercourse is based on a feeling that it threatens family life. Such a fear is far less frequently evoked by prostitution, which is less often regarded as a threat to society than as a blot upon it – a blot which it may be more possible to shut one's eyes to. Not only the personal fears of married women, but particularly the more impersonal fears for society, occur relatively seldom; here are two exceptions. The young wife of a Cardiff bus conductor is *"dead against it. My husband's been abroad, and the things he tells me make me mad. It wrecks homes."* And the 28 year old Birmingham housewife has similar fears:

> *"I reckon the prostitutes should all be shut up in a concentration camp. They are the ruin of many a happy marriage."*

For these women, prostitution has emerged from its water-tight compartment and constitutes a threat to their security and happiness. Similar signs of bitterness occasionally appear in the moral indignation of women who are jealous of the prostitute's well-being. A 47 year old Fulham housewife, for instance, part-time domestic worker, naively rejects prostitution:

> *"I'd sooner work than do that. I know a woman that does that, and she's got a new coat from knocking about with men, and she had the cheek to taunt me with having a shabby coat...."*

At the end of the interview this woman added spontaneously:

> *"My husband stays in and doesn't never go out, and won't let me go out. It's nothing but work, work, work; there's no enjoyment in life. All I do is go to the pictures once a week, and he doesn't like that; he's a lot older than me."*

Moral objections to prostitution are largely directed in this way against the prostitutes themselves. Except for a minority who regard her as unfortunate, the prostitute is usually felt by the morally disapproving to be hard, bad and degraded. She is even sometimes given responsibility for the system itself: *"I've got no time for that at all, a lot of them sort of women make men bad men"* said the elderly wife of a park-keeper.

To some extent the men who go to the prostitutes are included in the distaste and disapproval expressed about the women they frequent, but the bulk of moral feeling is directed against the latter. When the men are explicitly singled out for blame, practical criteria of physical need generally supersede moral ones: *"It's unnecessary. That's my plain view"* said a young Leeds factory worker. *"No man these days needs to go to a prostitute"*. And occasionally both partners are condemned to an equal extent as indulging in degrading sexual behaviour; sex that is exclusively physical is felt as usual to be not only distasteful but wrong. These are the points on which a headmaster, for instance, condemns prostitution:

> *"If we allow prostitution we admit that human beings are little higher than animals. The sexual act is humiliating unless it is accompanied by love."*

But on the whole the man's need of the prostitute is more widely recognised – as will be seen later – than the prostitutes' need to take to the street. Perhaps a less questionable objection, again based on practical grounds, is the risk of spreading V.D. This is one of the most frequent reasons for objecting to prostitution from the male rather than female angle; often, however, it is combined with a recommendation of medical control or of legalised brothels – suggesting that there are no intrinsic or moral objections to prostitution itself. A young Reigate motor mechanic, for instance, says candidly *"I don't go much on it myself. It spreads disease if it's not really looked after."*

The economic approach to prostitution is less frequent than the moral or medical one. Its usual form as a source of disapproval is the feeling that present day conditions provide plenty of legitimate work for everyone and the prostitute could keep off the streets if she really wished. But more often when people think in economic terms it is to excuse the prostitute rather than blame her for her profession. Even so both attitudes imply disapproval of prostitution itself; a 55 year old ship's rigger from Clydeside for instance, sympathises with the prostitute, but not with prostitution:

> *"It's the system that breeds it. It's no' for the love of sexual intercourse that a woman does that. It's necessity."*

From sympathising with the prostitute as driven into her job by economic forces, [it] is a small step to pitying her degradation. A fair-sized minority puts prostitution into its psychological and economic setting and, looking at it in this light, is sorry for the prostitute; a young Durham metal worker:

> *"From what I've seen of life, you needn't go to a prostitute the way things are now. But prostitutes are pretty bad. I think they are unlucky really. It's an affliction; to me it's like saying "What do you think about people who are T.B.""*

A prison officer's wife, thinking along similar lines, believes in prevention rather than cure:

> *"A lot depends on the way the children are brought up; their home life – everything should be done for the young people, likes of the Youth movement and one thing and another, to keep them off the street."*

Occasionally, on the other hand, a fairly reproachful and moralistic implication creeps into this type of semi-constructive view; a middle-aged Yorkshire housewife, for instance:

> *"Well, I deplore the fact that it exists. It needs spiritual uplift to get them out of it."*

Generally, objections to prostitution show something of the same pattern as attitudes to divorce and extra-marital relations. Moral disapproval is to varying extents tempered with humanitarian feeling and with at least partial understanding of the material and psychological exigencies which may not only drive women into prostitution, but also make it necessary for men to patronise the prostitutes. Sometimes this understanding becomes uppermost and prostitution is – usually with resignation – largely accepted. Altogether, one person in every six finds it, for one reason or another, possible to condone prostitution. This is almost always for purely practical reasons, almost no one goes out of his way to justify prostitution morally. Only occasionally is there an explicit suggestion that biological necessity renders prostitution morally justifiable [...].

> *"As regards to that, a man has a privilege to go with a woman if he wants to. It's kept under a cloak here and you have to go in a back street; but in Honolulu and the U.S.A. and Canada they've got licensed houses and no one interferes. I've been round them places."*

Just as the prostitute more often incurs moral disapproval than her client, so prostitution itself is usually condoned with the man in mind. Where prostitution is accepted it is usually on grounds of *masculine* human nature; many people say that prostitution always has existed and therefore must be expected to continue; nothing much can be done about it because it is a biological inevitability: *"If you're inclined that way, it's all right"*, said a Wigan window dresser. *"It's a very old profession, it doesn't harm anybody. It's always been, and it always will be."*

This fatalistic acceptance [....] of prostitution on the grounds that 'you can't change human nature' probably explains much of the futility that makes itself apparent in repudiation attitudes. Such fatalism is less common amongst the more educated – who are the more inclined to feel that prostitution would be eradicable under changed social and economic conditions. On the other hand, acceptance is often more positively reinforced by quite frequent references to special cases such as lechery, abnormality or marital discrepancy, in which recourse to prostitutes may be particularly necessary and inevitable; a Pontypool Pensioner agrees with prostitution on the grounds that *"my wife only wanted relationship once a week – she didn't think marriage was only for sex.".* Occasionally it is even felt that prostitution can happily supplement married life; a young Corporation Highways painter replied:

> *"In some ways it's a good thing. You get people who are not suited – but can make a happy family, apart from the matter of sex. So he goes elsewhere to satisfy his lust, and has a happy family at home. I think it would do good that way."*

Because satisfaction of sex desires is so often accepted as a necessity for men (not for women), a fairly frequent attitude amongst those who lean towards condoning prostitution is the feeling that it 'keeps the streets safe', protecting 'decent women' from assault. A Fulham tobacconist presented a slightly unusual aspect of this outlook when he said *"Prostitution is a good thing in respect that it keeps the straight girls in the right road.".* The uncontrollable male renders prostitution a biological inevitability. A similar reasoning is implicit in the suggestion that V.D. dangers make it necessary to legalise and medically control prostitution. References to the Continental system of legal brothels often contain more than a hint of wistfulness; it is more often women who regard the officially sanctioned brothel system as a way of dealing with an unpleasant but necessary evil – a Denbigh widow, for instance, diffidently:

> *"I abhor the thought of it, but I suppose it keeps ... Well, I suppose if there are licensed places like in France, it serves a purpose."*

Where the basic attitude to prostitution was one of disapproval, some sympathy for the prostitute occasionally emerged. Acceptance attitudes, on the other hand, are less often based on the prostitute's point of view; where they are it is usually to point out that prostitution may be a necessary means of livelihood for some women.

Generally, although the majority of people condemn prostitution, this is by no means always felt to be a straightforward moral issue. For very many people, particularly those who are no longer associated with any Church, expediency provides a more relevant criterion than the moral yardstick, and even humanitarian considerations:

> *"I don't know – sometimes I think they've not had a good set-up in life. Sometimes they'll point out to you a girl that's on the game and she doesn't look bad at all, you know what I mean – not a bad face. So I think there must be some good in them somewhere."*

Notes

1. Whatever the exact present-day frequency of brothels, it is at least certain that they are fewer and more furtive than they were 100 years ago. See Ivan Block, in his *Sexual Life in Great Britain*, (published by Alder, 1938) [....].

Part E, Sex and Life

Chapter Nine: The Psychology of Sex

Too complex and individual a matter for the social scientist, basic sex attitudes are justifiably a prerogative of the clinician and psycho-analyst. In this respect at least, all the social survey can reasonably attempt is a superficial coverage of general reactions to sex in a non-selected sample – a coverage which should make it possible to draw conclusions and generalise to the attitudes of the population as a whole. With this aim in view, we talked to people not only about the institutions of sex – an indirect means of exploring their feelings about sex itself – but also more boldly and directly about their reactions to its personal, rather than purely social, aspects.

One measure of what sex means to people is how much value they admit to it. Two out of every five, for instance, insist that it is possible to be happy 'without any form of sex life'. Men, young people, married people, the higher income (but not education) groups, and people who go to church irregularly or not at all, are more inclined to feel that sex is inseparable from happiness, whilst women, older and unmarried people, the lower income groups and regular churchgoers, tend to take the opposite view. The biggest difference is between men and women – not as in most other cases between churchgoers and non-churchgoers; two men in every five, and only one woman in every five, says that sex is indispensable to happiness. Of the whole 2,052 questioned:

33% said 'sexless' happiness was possible
8% said they could be happy without sex
32% said that 'sexless' happiness was impossible
9% said it depended on the individual
6% gave mixed views
3% gave miscellaneous views
9% were undecided or vague

Most people seem to take 'sex life' in this context to mean sexual intercourse; interpreting it in this way, opinion divided statistically into two similarly sized groups, one denying that sex is essential to happiness, the other regarding it as indispensable. Qualitatively, however, there is a less clear-cut division of outlook; feeling is seldom very strong on either side, and terms of reference are in either case usually practical rather than moral. But to some extent people who insist that life can be happy without sex tend to be rather the more vehement and moralistic in their views. Sometimes, for instance, there is a suggestion that happiness ought to be possible without sex; a 47 year old boat-builder, 8 years married, said scornfully, *"There's more important things in life than sex, though you mightn't think so to hear some men talk"*, and a 68 year old Exeter labourer insists:

> *"People who cannot be happy without sex are more beasts than men. It is the happiness of the union that matters. My wife was ill for 18 months after our first baby was born, and after that she had a dropped womb. But we worked things out accordingly, my wife and I, and it did not affect our happiness."*

The special nature of this man's marital position may well explain much of his unusually bitter feeling. But although his bitterness is unusual, his suggestion that people who cannot do without sex are somehow morally at fault is much less rare. Like him, many people feel not only that sex desires can be deflected into non-sexual channels, but also that such deflection ought to be achieved where necessary. Occasionally there is even a suggestion that asceticism is a desirable end in itself; *"If they love each other they ought to put sex on one side"*, said the middle-aged wife of a Pontypool workingman, *"Sex isn't the only thing in life. That's how I look at it."*.

But most of this larger group who play sex down do so more simply and tentatively, and without any apparent reference to morality. A middle-aged spinster, for instance, says she has had no sexual experience but is *"quite a happy woman myself, you can make yourself happy if you have other interests"*. A 55 year-old bachelor (a Glasgow labourer) is *"as happy as a bee myself, and I'm not caring a hoot about sex. I suppose it will be different with people of different natures."* A young married woman thinks in more academic terms: *"It wouldn't worry me if I wasn't married and hadn't a boy friend"*. And a middle-aged housewife, who first heard about sex 'not in a nice way' and says that 'in a way' she is getting what she wants from life – (*"I don't go out now, but I've got the children"*) finds it easy to do without sex:

> *"I can be happy without sex, it's only duty for me now, and it's the same with my husband."*

Whatever their assessment of the importance of sex, not many people explicitly express really bitter or moralistic views; this is particularly rare amongst those who attach most importance and value to sex, when it is usually largely a result of exceptional circumstances. A middle-aged factory labourer, for instance, unhappily married:

> *"No, I can't live happily without sex; and the wife who says, 'Hurry up, I'm tired', wants her ears boxing ... yes, sex can be unpleasant – as I've just said when the wife is unwilling it makes a man feel like a sexual brute."*

More usual amongst the group who insist on sex for happiness is a touch of scorn and sexual pride. The young Welsh wife of a garage man feels that *"it has an effect on people's minds to do without. I mean you see these single women busying themselves with their jobs, trying to achieve frustration"*. And a middle-aged Newcastle factory worker explains:

> *"I don't know, you can see women that's never been happy, and men that's never had a woman. And they look as if they're going seedy, they have that green and mouldy look".*

Even more frequent is the view that sex is indispensable to a full life because it is a natural human function. A middle-aged factory worker says *"That's what you really marry for, people say it is love but it is really sex"*. And a Scottish porter regards it as *"only natural for a human being, just like it is for the birds and the beasts"*. 'That's natural' is a recurring theme, and not only in answer to this question. Sex knowledge is felt to grow 'naturally', birth control flies in the face of 'natural' sex relations, prostitution, extra-marital relations are felt to be inevitable because of 'human nature'. Later it will also be seen that sex is often felt not to be wrong, unpleasant or harmful – but simply 'natural'. Nevertheless, although the 'naturalness' of sex is so frequently recognised, it is often only within the conventionally specified limits: sex may be natural, but only in so far as it is also reasonably orthodox – particularly only in so far as it occurs within the context of marriage. *"After marriage it's more or less a natural activity"*, said a 34 year old fitter's wife, *"There's something sacred about it"*. And a young Manchester housewife feels that *"sex life comes with marriage, that's all. I've never thought of it except as part of marriage – but in marriage it helps to bind you together"*.

Extending this attitude a bit further, some people not only identify sex with marriage, but also with marriage and children; in this sense of its family setting, sex is felt to be natural and essential to happiness. Not merely sex, but family life is indispensable. A 58 year old Ayrshire baker, for instance:

> *"When a man and a woman come to a certain time in life, and they want a place to settle down together, and live as man and wife, that's natural".*

This conception of sex and family life as almost interchangeable concepts is behind much street sample feeling that sex is necessary to happiness. And sometimes, amongst those holding the opposite view, a refusal to consider sex in anything but its narrowest form is the reason for regarding it as not strictly necessary. *"Sex doesn't give you happiness, only excitement"*, said a retired teacher, a husband of 45 years standing. And a young Nottingham housewife-machinist explains *"Some people are more sexual than others, that's the trouble, and some people in need of love and comfort mistake that for need of sex"*.

Others take a more fatalistic view. For them, the 'naturalness' of sex is limited less by convention than by the vagaries of personal make-up. A 45 year old housekeeper:

> *"Sex is part of my nature. Some people are born sexual and others are not"*

Belief in the essential relation between sex and happiness tends to increase with income. Partly a reflection of this relationship, more than half of the Mass-Observation National Panel group agreed that sex is vital for happiness; but once again the basic manner of approach to the problem is much the same. Fundamentally there seems to be a similar practical emphasis on psychological and biological effects rather than on moral criteria; the man-in-the-street has apparently absorbed much of the modern psychological outlook – but the middle class man has a greater capacity for expressing this in semi-psychological terms, and with the added confidence conferred by this capacity. The concepts of 'sublimation' and 'repression' in particular recur amongst the Panel replies as frequently as the term 'natural' in the street. *"Plenty of people are happy without any sex life, but are probably unconsciously repressed"*, says one young research chemist, for instance, and a salesman believes in sublimation up to a point:

> *"One can be seemingly happy in the sublimation of the sex drive, is one really happy without normal sexual satisfaction?"*

Generally the concept of sublimation seems to have less sway than realisation of the neurotic effects of [....] over-sex repression and the all-importance of the sex drive. This acceptance of the individual's need of a direct sex outlet is probably, as usual, the direction in which popular opinion is drifting; conventional limits placed to the indispensability of sex would seem to be widening; unmarried need of a sex outlet begins to be recognised, even if the outlet is only of the mildest kind. *"Dancing, or taking a girl to the pictures"*, suggested one young draughtsman.

But narrowing or not, the conventional limits remain. Sexual activity is hedged in by anxieties, inhibitions and taboos, restrictions which we set out tentatively to explore. We asked people three questions, deliberately framed in such a way as to dig out as much as possible of existing moral disapproval, personal disgust, fears, dislikes and limits and barriers to sex. They were asked whether they thought that sex was 'in any way' wrong, unpleasant or harmful; each time a recurring reply was, quite simply, 'sex is natural'. In spite of the lead inherent in the questions, only 26% agreed that sex could be wrong, 48% that it could be in any way unpleasant, and 60% that it might be harmful. Often our suggestions came up against an indignant wall of resistance. *"Sexual intercourse? That's not wrong at all. How can it be? It produces children"*, reasoned one elderly man, a retired teacher, by no means unrepresentative in his views.

Sex is a natural function, common to all, universal and eternal, biologically essential to continuing human life – these are constantly recurring views. Religious justifications are quite often brought in to provide additional emphasis; a young Methodist woman, for instance, insisted that *"sex isn't wrong, it's created by God"*. But on the whole people who go to church are rather more suspicious of sex than any others of our sub-groups. Regular churchgoers are only slightly more inclined to accept the suggestion that sex is indispensable to happiness – but to a more marked degree they suspect it of being, in some circumstances at least, wrong or unpleasant. Other group differences are slighter and less consistent.

Very few people express any fundamental objection to sex in itself – although we did come across a few such cases, some of which have already been quoted. A labouring class house-wife, for instance, says that *"men are like that, and we women have to put up with it in order to have children"*, and a young Welsh student regards sex as unpleasant because *"I like to regard women as beautiful"*. A middle aged working class housewife thinks:

> *"sex is very unpleasant. My husband says I'm not human. If I'd known what it was like before I got married, I never would have married at all."*

And another labourer's wife:

> *"Intercourse is not right, really, is it? Not even if you are married .... Sex isn't very nice, to a woman it's not very nice. It is sort of unpleasant to a girl, it's not very nice at all... Yes, it can be harmful, it can ruin a woman's inside as easy as pie, ruin any girl's innards, intercourse can ..."*

This housewife, although a non churchgoer, is consistent in her condemnation of almost every aspect of sex – divorce, for instance is a 'sin against the Lord Almighty', prostitutes should be locked up, extra-marital relations should be legislated against, and standards of sex morality are deteriorating. One partial clue to her hostile attitude to the world in general may be her unhappy home background (*"My father used to drink a terrible lot, always coming back full of beer he was"*). But in any case, like the others to whom sex is intrinsically undesirable, she is exceptional. For the vast majority, explicit objections to sex are applied only to certain cases of infringement of conventional ethics

– to extra-marital intercourse for instance, to which 13% spontaneously objected. The matter-of-fact way in which most people mention this marriage bar, moreover, suggests that it would come up far more often if many more were not taking it for granted; it has already been seen that asked directly about this, as many as two thirds of the whole sample disapproved. This is the most important of the conventional limits that people set to the natural 'rightness' of sex. Others emerge only very occasionally. Here are total results to the question on whether sex is wrong:

76% said it was not wrong
13% said it was wrong outside marriage
2% said it was wrong if overdone
1% said it was wrong if abnormal
1% said it was wrong if lacking in affection
2% said vaguely it could be wrong
1% said it was wrong for miscellaneous reasons
4% had no opinion

Moral condemnation aimed at extra-marital relations overshadows all the other conventional barriers – in so far as surface opinion goes, at least. But sexual taboos are as likely to emerge indirectly as directly, and ways in which people suspect sex of unpleasantness or harmfulness may often be indications of moral restrictions at a less conscious level. One person in every five, for instance, particularly thinks that sex would be harmful if overdone; and one in twenty-five has similar ideas about its unpleasantness. These fears of too-frequent sexual activity tend to show at least a suggestion of conventional morality and irrationality. And something of the same moral origin is also probably present in the reasoning of the one in twenty who say that affectionless sex would be unpleasant. *"You would have to be very attached to someone before it would seem to be pleasant"*, said a middle-aged widowed shop keeper. Thinking along something of the same lines, similar proportions, men and women equally, object to sex where both partners are not entirely willing. The 39 year old wife a Yorkshire plumber for instance:

> *"It is unpleasant sometimes. When you're tired out after a washing day, and you don't want it. You don't want the man then"*

Psychiatrists and sexologists find it difficult to agree as to what sexual behaviour is normal and abnormal and are often wary of setting standards at all. The man in the street is less cautious of committing himself. Although he seldom specifies exactly what he means by abnormal sex behaviour, he quoted abnormality occasionally not only as wrong, but also as unpleasant and harmful. There are two dimensions to sex normality – first the nature and second the frequency of sexual activity. It is for the most part along lines of the first that sex is felt to be unpleasant – and of the second that it is felt to be harmful. Both kinds of reference tend to be equally shadowy. Some people refer vaguely to 'What you read in the papers'. Others, like this middle aged Welshman, say that abnormality is *"doing what you shouldn't in intercourse"*. And too frequent intercourse is felt to be physically bad for people. *"It wears people out too much of it"* said a middle-aged labourer, and a 30 year old housewife feels that *"it must pull your weight down or cause something if you have too much"*. Sometimes psychological and mental, even moral ill-effects are mentioned. *"Sex can distort people's minds, if it is preyed upon"*, said the middle-aged wife of a Denbigh shop-keeper, adding apologetically *"You know what I mean"*. And a 47 year old factory worker:

> *"Well, sex can harm you if you let it get too strong a hold on you. It's like drink, it becomes a vice."*

But sometimes – as in these cases just quoted – it is doubtful whether people are thinking in terms of too much overt sex activity, or too much preoccupation with sex on a mental or emotional level. For this 39 year old spinster, however, it is clear that the difficulty is a matter of temptation alone: *"It can be harmful if it's too much thought about"*, she said *"and reading the wrong kind of book can give people immoral thoughts"*.

Fear of sex 'getting a hold on you' seems to be the focus of a considerable amount of anxiety. Past Mass-Observation surveys on smoking, drinking and gambling have shown similar inhibitory fears in each of those fields. And in the sexual sphere indulgence beyond the unspecified normal standard of frequency is felt to have all the ill-effects of the unknown and unprecedented. This anxiety may have a two-way relation to the popular insistence on regarding sex as a non-essential to happiness: sex is kept under control not only by decrying and avoiding too-frequent sex relations, but also by playing down its importance. And both symptoms of uneasiness are probably derived from moral and religious roots, just as they are more obviously related to opinion on the more clear-cut subjects of unmarried sex, birth-control and prostitution. Behind it all there seems to lurk the suspicion that sex indulged in for its own sake is wrong – and as such also unpleasant, harmful, and needful of control by accepted standards of normality. *"Sex can be wrong – it could be mis-used"* said a 35 year old commercial traveller, a church-goer, who proceeds to explain, *"To enjoy it for the excitement rather than just the need is wrong"*.

Other sources of uneasiness about sex appear much less frequently. Replies to the question whether sex is wrong have already been given in statistical form. Here are similarly tabulated data on the harmfulness and unpleasantness of sex. It must be remembered that none of these individual reasons were enquired about specifically.

6% said that sex could not be unpleasant
6% said it was unpleasant if not mutually willing

5% " " " " if lacking affection
4% " " " " if abnormal
4% " " " " if overdone
3% " " " " if there were risk of VD
2% " " " " outside marriage
1% " " " " in ill-health
1% " " " " if it were brutal

[And also]
[....] said sex could not be harmful
20% said sex could be harmful if overdone
11% " if there was risk of VD
3% " if abnormal
3% " in ill health
2% " outside marriage
1% " if not mutually willing
1% " if it were brutal

These were the main contingencies uppermost in people's minds. Results suggest that, apart from the moral bar against sex relations outside marriage, most of the top-level sexual anxieties and taboos concern either the normalities of frequencies or nature of intercourse, the affection with which sexual activities are accompanied, or, more practically, the risk of V.D. This last fear occurs particularly amongst young unmarried men, [....] who explicitly mention it as one of the ways in which sex can harm people who are 'not careful'. But V.D. anxieties would seem to be more prevalent than they at first sight appear; references are often oblique and hesitant – 'those diseases' are mentioned more often than the more outright 'V.D.'. *"Diseases and all sorts of things"*, said the 35 year old wife of a Welsh garage manager, cautiously.

But uneasiness about sex manifests itself mainly in setting limits of married legitimacy, of nature and frequency. Education is inclined to decrease insistence on the marriage limit and to increase insistence on keeping it within the bounds of 'normal' nature. Comparison of the street sample as a whole with the middle-class Panel group puts these differences, as it were, under a magnifying glass. Thinking their replies out in the leisure of their own homes, the Panel group are far more inclined to think of ways in which sex may be wrong, unpleasant or harmful (note 1); their replies also tend to take a more impersonal form and to be more elaborated and clearly defined than those of people interviewed in the street who are, inevitably, more or less surprised into giving unconsidered their views. But it is not extramarital relations but sex of an abnormal nature, affectionless sex, over-preoccupation with sex, and over-frequent indulgence, that emerge as the chief focal points of Panel anxiety [....]. Once again psychological terms and concepts occur very frequently. The following questionnaire extracts have been chosen as fairly typical examples of these considered views from a group above average in intelligence and education.

Is sex in any way wrong?

"This is an absurd question. Sex, my sex, or yours, is a fact. It cannot be wrong, any more than can the colour of my hair; it's there." (27 year old man, publishing office).

"How can a natural function be wrong? It can be used wrongly" (48 year old journalist).

"I feel that it is wrong if used merely to satisfy desire; if the element of love or tenderness is lacking then it seems to me that the elements of viciousness and sadism begin to appear." (28 year old professional woman, unmarried).

"Yes, over-indulgence, inconsiderate sensuality, sadism, and in all sorts of circumstances." 55 year old museum director.

Can sex be in any way unpleasant?

"Yes, certainly. If perverted or mischievous or underhand, or hopelessly frustrated, or hopelessly promiscuous." (29 year old man, publishing worker).

"Yes, when it is abnormal, or if the persons are ignorant, or have a 'warped view' of what sex really is." (22 year old police sergeant).

"If exaggerated in importance, and mixed up with unconnected things – so that it becomes inartistically obtrusive and obviously obsessional." (32 year old shipping clerk).

"When perverted as in sadism or masochism." (25 year old research chemist).

Only occasionally does a really personal note creep in amongst this group: A middle-aged housewife, for instance, who describes herself as a *"domestic servant in husband's house"*:

"I think sex is a dirty and objectionable form of procreation, but cannot be helped. It is unpleasant in every way for me."

Can sex harm people in any way?

"Through lack of knowledge or the wrong approach". (31 year old telegraph engineer)

> *"Over-indulgence, extreme sex behaviour, sadism and masochism, can weaken and destroy a person's health and character".* (40 year old company director)

> *"By becoming an obsession and diverting the boy or girl from his chosen work. It does interfere so! Too much indulgence is coarsening and weakening."* (49 year old housewife)

> *"Excessive indulgence will definitely weaken a man in time. Illicit sexual practices always run the risk of V.D. Excess of any sort leads to neurosis."* (34 year old school master)

> *"If they come to regard it as something nasty or unpleasant, I should say that it could cause much alarm, worry and nervous strain."* (23 year old clerk)

There is no doubt but that uneasiness about sexual preoccupation and over-indulgence is at least equally frequent in this educated and semi-professional Panel group as in the street sample as a whole. But the Panel has another fear to counter-balance this one: they are alert to the ill-effects of the opposite extreme, afraid not only of sex becoming too important but also that it may be denied its due: sex, they say, may be harmful if too rigorously denied, and 'repression' becomes for them a bogey of almost equal dimensions with 'indulgence' and 'lust'. *"Too much restraint, I think that causes harm to one's nervous system"*, says a 44 year old estate clerk, and a young research engineer sees a double danger:

> *"One can definitely have over-indulgence. And sex-repression unexpressed in other directions is often a cause of mental, psychological and physical trouble".*

Generally it seems fairly clear that people's approach to sex tends to be limited not only by their intentness on doing what they regard as socially 'correct', but also by anxieties and fears, particularly fears of transgressing the bounds of 'normality', and which may be all the stronger for their vagueness. A welter of half-absorbed, half-understood psychological concepts, particularly the superficially conflicting concepts of sublimation and repression, adds to the confusion. And to some extent these lurking anxieties and inhibitions underline the point stressed in earlier chapters, that people are trouble by what is possibly a deep-rooted conflict between on the one hand their acceptance of the natural inevitability of sex, and on the other the tradition, founded possibly in religious asceticism, that sex for its own sake is lust and wrong (note 2).

Notes

1 Only one Panel member in eleven denies that sex can be unpleasant and one in every seventeen its potential harmfulness. One in every two – compared with three-quarters of the street sample – insists that sex is not in any way wrong.
[2 The chapter concludes at this point, but is apparently unfinished.]

Chapter Ten: Sexual Morality and the Position Today

There is no doubt that people today are confused about the oughts of sexual behaviour. It may be that such confusion is greater today than it has been in the past – but in the absence of early comparative material this is impossible to judge; and partial break-away from the other absolute standards of sex morality make it at least likely that ideas generally are less clean-cut than they once were. The individual is to some extent inevitably left to develop new standards for himself – and the confusion is increased by the haphazard nature of such individual thinking, a half-aware accumulation of often conflicting tenets rather than conscious decision making. Pulpit, surgery, birth control clinic, novelty, confessional, street corner, the film picture of the psychiatrist's consulting room with its mid-century prestige and glamour, all contribute to a conglomeration of ill-sorted ideas, half absorbed, half understood, often half-rejected. One outcome of a social survey is almost invariably realisation of the context to which people's ideas are governed less by logic than by feeling; not even the social psychiatrist can be more confused than the individual units of the masses he studies.

Confusion is in some ways unanswered by people's awareness that not only abstract standards but actual behaviour is changing. Ideas of normality to some extent govern ideas of morality, and uncertainty as to what other people do may make it more difficult than ever for the man in the street to decide just what is normal and what is not. At the beginning of our questionnaire we introduced the subject of sex by asking people whether they though 'standards of sex morality today are getting better or worse or remaining about the same' – and why. Most people judged moral standards by behaviour and nearly every second person, looking at the question in this light, said standards were going down.

Of all the 2,052 people questioned by Mass-Observation:

44% said standards were declining
29% said they were much the same as ever
17% said they were improving
10% were undecided or vague

Age seems to be the strongest factor influencing people on these points, even stronger than the usually most powerful factor of church-going; on the whole the young take an optimistic view and the old a pessimistic one. 56% of all the young people under 25 say either that standards are improved or unaltered, compared with only 31% of the over 45s, just over half of whom say standards have deteriorated. To some extent attitudes seem to resolve themselves into the traditional head-shaking over the younger generation. The young adult even blames the adolescent:

> *"Adults' sexual behaviour is all right, but the juveniles is a bit scandalous. Young girls going for walks in the dark parts or in the woods. I've seen them. Why I've had them screaming out as I passed by.... If they go walking in the dark with their lads they know what to expect, and they get it."* (23 year old labourer's handyman, Blackburn)

Churchgoing seems to exercise only a slight influence on attitudes to present-day morality – weekly churchgoers are a little inclined to be more pessimistic than irregular or non-churchgoers. Our distinct and selected sample of clergymen, however, showed an opinion pattern as usual very different from that of the average; three clergymen out of every five felt that moral standards were declining, compared with two in every five of the street sample. Quite clearly churchgoers are less inclined to absorb the opinion of their religious leaders on this score than they are on most other aspects of sexual morality – extra-marital relations, divorce or birth control, for instance.

Middle class people and people with more education and money are also more inclined to take a favourable view of changing sexual morality than the financially and socially less well-off; and this difference is again reflected and pin-pointed in the views of teachers, doctors – and of Mass-Observation's National Panel. As might be expected, the National Panel – representing to some extent 'free-thinking' people – are the champions of sexual freedom and knowledge, and are most inclined to take a favourable view of changes in sexual morality; three in every five of them feel that moral standards are improving or else remaining unchanged, compared with:

one teacher in every two
two doctors in every five
just over two in every five of the street sample
and one clergyman in every four

Education quite clearly influences people towards accepting present-day developments in sexual morality and behaviour as at least no change for the worse. Income differences show that the poorer people are most inclined to feel that standards are deteriorating. Perhaps this social difference is related to the fact that pessimism is most common amongst the section of discontented people who say they are not getting what they want from life.

Marriage, on the other hand, seems to have little effect, and differences between men and women are negligible. Generally views of morality seem partially to depend on education and to some extent on the strength of church-ties, but to an even greater extent they remain a matter of generation. But irrespective of their individual background and whether they feel moral standards are changing for the better or the worse, most people agree at least that the outward forms of sexual behaviour are changing towards greater frankness, and freedom; the question in many people's minds is whether this is a desirable development, and also whether it implies a corresponding change in moral standards themselves. The majority of those who feel that standards are the same make a major point of this possibility that behaviour is remaining constant even though what was formerly concealed is now openly discussed. A 27 year old milk roundsman, for instance, says *"It's no worse than it used to be when everything was hidden"*, and a woman farmer, 52, from Tadcaster,

> *"I think things are much as they always were. Well, I just base that on what I see in the neighbourhood. It's only more obvious now. It used to be more on the furtive side."*

Those who think standards are getting better also base many of their arguments on this same point, the increasing knowledge of sex and increasing freedom in sexual behaviour; to them these things may be seen either as causes or as results of improvement. This opinion is rather commoner amongst women than amongst men, perhaps because recent freedom and knowledge have been much to women's benefit. Here, for instance, is the opinion of a middle-aged Clydeside housewife:

> *"Young people are getting more enlightened – not so narrow as when we were youngsters."* (wife of an insurance agent, 51, Greenock)

The other major group amongst the optimists thinks less of long-term changes than in terms of a war-time slackening of standards which they think are now tightening up again, and to the[m], apparently, pre-war norm was [....]:

> *"Standards are going up as far as I can see. The war is over and we're getting settled down now."* (foundry furnace-man, aged 25, Leeds)

> *"Oh, not any worse at all, better now the war's over. There was a lot of talk about what went on then – all these men in the country – a girl in town had a little half caste and there were a lot of black babies in Manchester. But you couldn't call that normal. Now things have settled down. Well, I shouldn't say they're any worse at all ... I think we're all right here. And you can see for yourself, young people settling down sensibly together."* (Publican's wife, aged 54, Rochdale)

People who think moral standards are improving are inclined to base their views in this way, on observation. As many as one in every six, on the other hand, of those who take a pessimistic view of present-day morality derive their opinions either explicitly or inexplicitly from what they read in the papers. This is particularly true of young people and women; one quarter of the pessimists amongst women mention newspaper reports. A 39 year old (331) housewife, wife of a civil servant said:

"The News of the World is evidence enough"

and two other women:

"Oh things are definitely worse. Well, look what you see around you. And in the papers – all these attacks. You're almost afraid to go out." (46 year old butcher's wife, Leeds)

"I think there is far more sex erring than there used to be" (28 year old (244) domestic worker, separated from husband)

Newspaper resistance is much stronger amongst those who believe morality is growing better; this group often says *"Of course, you can't believe what you see in the papers"*. Other Mass-Observation material, tracing reactions to newspapers from the beginning of the war onwards, indicates that up to a few years ago much scepticism was slowly increasing, and that the last few years have at least maintained that increased level of distrust. The beginnings of such scepticism are occasionally seen amongst those who on the whole still have faith in the [newspapers]:

"Things are getting worse. There's more cases in the news. Of course it is possible that in the past there wasn't so much publicity, but just as much immorality – but on the whole I don't think that it is so." (40 year old engineering draughtsman, Manchester)

And a few suggest that newspaper reports not only reflect declining morals, but even help to cause them:

"Standards are getting worse. Well, you can't pick up a paper without something in it about sex. My little girl makes me blush, she asks so many questions which never occurred to me at her age." (39 year old London woman, separated from her husband, living with an engineer, himself separated from his wife.)

But pessimistic opinions are not all based on hearsay; one in every five claim personal observation and experience of the behaviour of young people, as well as an additional one in six who say they blame the women and young people. Young women are especially liable to come in for criticism. As one elderly Scot said sadly:

> *"Years ago you could tell a respectable lassie by the way she dressed. Now you can't tell at all. They all dress alike, they paint and powder the same."*

But condemnation of the younger generation is frequently combined with criticism of the upbringing they have received. Lack of discipline is a common cause for complaint; one in every seventeen, men especially, point to some example of wrong or inadequate influence:

> *"Oh things are worse. I see so much of it. I can see it going on with the young people in pubs, night after night. Young girls waiting outside until all hours, and then making off with the men up the dark streets. It's because the parents have lost control over their children."* (45 year old wages clerk, Shrewsbury)

> *"Standards are getting worse. It's as plain as anything to see. Look at the way the dance halls are filled every day. There's no discipline in young people these days."* (68 year old pensioner, Birmingham)

One in every nine, especially, were blaming the decline in sexual morality to the man and – particularly – to the American 'invasion', of British towns and villages; but these are the more optimistic of the pessimists – the war time upheaval may have had only temporary effects. An (622) elderly housewife says:

> *"Things are worse. Goodness me, you never heard of the things years ago that we do today. It's due to the war and fellows getting wild."*

To the 'man in the street', sexual behaviour seems to be growing, whether for better or worse, more free and undisguised. If he thinks this is an undesirable development a different choice of terms puts it into a different light, labelling it as loose, blatant and uncontrolled; this varying interpretation of the same facts is especially apparent amongst the views of our samples of doctors, teachers, clergymen, so called 'leaders of opinion'. To clergymen, particularly, greater freedom and openness tends not to mean a changing moral criterion but a break-away from the only true Christian standards of morality:

> *"The change taking place is away from morality. Sexual relations are regarded more as a matter of personal feeling and an inclination of the moment."* (42 year old clergyman)

And a 73 year old Church of England clergyman, regretfully:

"People speak more openly about sex. Many think it a matter of private judgement. There is no absolute standard any more."

To most clergymen, standards are becoming 'lower' in as much as they are departing from the accepted morality of the Church; few see the question in the light of standards changing in kind rather than degree. The few who feel that morality is improving stress the decline in furtiveness as a desirable development, and welcome what they construe as a more pliable and positive attitude to sex. This exceptional young clergyman puts both points of view:

"Instead of sticking to a true and lasting principle, people are in the main treating sexual morality as a matter of personal convenience and inclination. This is for the better, if sex is seen to be in itself a good thing, nothing to feel guilty about; but for the worse if this attitude results in a loss of sense of responsibility in sexual matters. Freedom without responsibility is license or anarchy."

To this clergyman, a breakdown of absolute morality does not necessarily mean no morality at all. Even so, most clergymen appear to think in terms of a lowering morality, and conceptions of changing standards are on the whole rather more common amongst doctors and teachers, and much more frequent in the views of Mass-Observation's National Panel. A middle-aged schoolmaster, for instance, looks at the present-day phases as a step towards a new morality, more or less historical, an inevitability:

"People are more self-indulgent and unrestrained by future responsibility, or by doctrine. This change is for the better in that it is dynamic, not static, a development stage in moral values."

And a doctor welcomes increasing freedom:

"Sex problems are discussed more freely amongst young people. There are fewer taboos in the relations between young people of opposite sex. The relationship is more 'natural'".

Even so, not more than one doctor in five and one teacher in three believes that moral standards are changing for the better. Increasing sexual freedom is far more often decried than welcomed, and even amongst teachers (most inclined to welcome the spread of knowledge and increase in discussion), laxity is a more frequently recurring term than frankness. Relaxing restrictions are felt to constitute a threat to family life; a young married doctor, for instance:

"I think the change is rather in the increasing laxity of morality of all types, not only sexually and in the general belief and realisation that

*public opinion is much less strict in its judgement on the back slider
... There can be no doubt that the changes are for the worse. They tend
to undermine and destroy the family unit (see the divorce court).
They do not increase the sum total of human happiness. And the consequent lack of security and loss of value have a wholly detrimental
effect upon the future generation – they are undermining the moral
fibre of the nation."*

Clergymen are very conscious of disintegrating values, doctors, teachers, and
population as a whole are less so, and members of Mass-Observation's
National Panel most of all are inclined to look at the present situation
unemotionally as a historical phase – and as such to accept it, if not as an
improvement on the past, at least as no symptom of a lowering morality.
Panel attitudes pin-point this comparatively philosophical view of morality:
the relative weaknesses of their ties with the Church, as well as their custom-
ary tendency to take a social view of problems generally, may help them to
take up a comparatively impersonal stand-point. On this particular score one
in every three insists that moral standards are unchanged, and an additional
one in every four of them feels that standards are changing for the better. The
usual emphasis is either on the absence of any fundamental change, or else,
where change is conceded, on the suggestion that it is a change in kind rather
than degree:

*"Standards are freer, though not necessarily worse. People are adopt-
ing a more material attitude to life, and are questioning the conventions once accepted."* (22 year old research chemist.)

*"Everything is more open and above board, folk talk sex today. Fifty
years ago it was taboo, but just as powerful, I believe. Human nature
has altered little – boys and girls have more freedom, war always
bears its mark. No, generally, I do not think the standards are lower."*
(51 year old schoolmaster)

And an elderly engineer claims to speak from experience:

*"I should say standards are no worse than 40 years ago. As a young
man I had no difficulty in having a girl friend, and I know that the
young men of the present-time find things just as easy."*

This ability to look at the situation in its historical context of both past and
future, rather than attach to it the heightened importance of the isolated
moment, is to some extent the key to the relative absence of emotionality
amongst the National Panel group. Doctors and teachers and the street sample show the same tendency to a less pronounced degree, but clergymen, in
contrast, cling more to the present and past, resentful of any change. There

seems, however, to be little doubt that behaviour is changing – if only out-wardly, and in the long run attitudes and standards are bound to change too. The pronounced tendency for young people to take a more tolerant view of present-day morality suggests that this is the direction in which opinion is moving. [That is,] towards the conception, more prevalent amongst not only younger people but also the middle classes, and pin-pointed in Panel opinion, of a new morality rather than a lowered one, a morality which not only allows more open sexual behaviour, and discussion, but also makes allowance for deviation from what it still to some extent regards as a desirable standard of monogamy; and finally shows some signs of passing moral judgement accord-ing to individual and social criteria (taking into account, for instance, the feel-ings involved in extra-marital relations, and the question of whether or not such relations injure anyone beyond the two strictly concerned) rather than judging morality according to purely absolute standards.

Some idea of what is happening to morality can be gained by compari-son of the attitudes of one group with those of another; comparison of the behaviour of different groups is likely to clarify the position still further. Working to this end, we made a study of the outward pattern of sexual behav-iour in two towns of quite different character; the first a small Cathedral city, and the second an industrial town and seaport with a population nearly twice as large again and predominantly working class in character. We called the first 'Churchtown' and the second 'Steeltown'. At the level of official statis-tics, the difference between the two is not striking in proportion to the size of the population. Steeltown convictions for drunkenness are least ten times as many as in Churchtown – but convictions for soliciting and brothel keeping are almost down to nil in either case. Steeltown in 1948 produced just over three times as many cases of V.D. as Churchtown, and in 1946 – when such statistics were last available – twice as many illegitimate births; but if these figures are considered in relation to the size of the population, much of the apparent differences fade out, leaving a picture of two areas, which, on the face of it, are not too dissimilar.

But the key phrase is on the face of it. In qualities that cannot be mea-sured statistically, the two towns are very different. In Churchtown, the pat-tern of overt sexual behaviour is on the whole restrained, conventional and unsophisticated, whereas public behaviour in the pubs, dance halls, parks and streets of Steeltown tends to be much more free and openly provocative. Quite apart from the difference in incidence of prostitution, already dis-cussed in Chapter 8, ordinary relations between the sexes are very different. This contrast is apparent even in the attitudes of the two sets of town officials. Here, for instance is the official picture of Churchtown, expressed informally by the town's executives; the Chief Constable finds very little to worry about:

"There are no known prostitutes operating at all ... there is certainly
no public love-making going on of any description, not even in a mid-
dle sort of way. During the war we used to be bothered with couples

in shop doorways after nightfall, but all that has stopped now. The people here are not the kind to do that. There are no bad spots ... Soliciting may be practised in a limited way in the public houses, but it is doubtful. The river banks are not a problem, we keep a watchful eye on them in the summer and nothing resembling 'vice' is practised there. Yes, we find the usual collection of young lovers on a fine evening but that is to be expected. ... The dance halls are very well conducted and since the war there has been no trouble in there ... there is very little excessive drinking..."

But at a less official level, talking with a P.C. on the beat, produced a slightly less cheerful picture:

"Churchtown's really a very quite place. There's not much trouble now. It was hectic during the war, of course, but even then it never got out of hand ... night duty was the time. You'd get the shop doorway's full, and you'd have to clear them out. But it's all right now. After half past ten there's nothing doing at all. Sometimes you can do a whole duty at night without seeing a soul after 11 o'clock. There's a few hobos hang out at C... Corner, but we shift them on and they don't cause trouble. There's only one part of the town where you get any real immorality, that's those common lodging houses back of ....; but they're very quiet about it so the police don't trouble them. They don't mind much who they take in, and I think all the girls who pick up fellows take them to these houses. No, they're all amateurs, we had prostitutes during the war, but they were mostly from out of town, they came after the Americans."

"Nothing after 11 o'clock", "But they're very quiet about it.", "It was hectic during the war, of course", "They were mostly from out of town" – the picture already emerges of post war quietude, out of town scapegoats, and the policy of laissez-faire so long as everyone keeps sufficiently quiet. The Secretary of the Marriage Guidance Society tells the same story of small town absence of open immorality:

"I've no way of knowing how sexual morality compares with other areas, except from newspaper information, but I think there has been a considerable loosening in the last ten years. ... But now I imagine Churchtown stands quite high in comparison with other places. That may be because there is always less immorality in a community where everyone knows everyone else, at least open immorality. And in many respects Churchtown is still a county town with country traditions even though it is in the process of being industrialised ... the loosening of moral standards isn't really very serious. I imagine it's no more than a general tendency amongst young people to assert themselves

and mix more freely. There is no obvious immorality worth speaking about ... Of course, my opinion is based only on fairly casual observation and hearsay. Immorality is not the sort of thing that one can discuss with certainty, because it is so very difficult to know what is beneath the surface."

It is difficult to know what lies beneath the surface; but it is significant that Churchtown depths seem particularly impenetrable. A woman J.P. said *"I wouldn't dare to attempt to assess the standards of sexual morality in Churchtown, it is an impossible question for me to answer"*. But by no means all the town's officials are so cautious, or so aware of private depths from which public figures may be [the] first to be excluded. An outsider would need to live in Churchtown for many months at least before he was sufficiently assimilated into the local life to assess the deeper level of behaviour; but even with the limited time at our disposal we were in a rather better position, in our anonymity, than high-ranking town officials. Even so, an official report of the moral picture did not show it in a very different light; 'immorality' quite clearly does exist, but furtively, and in so far as it is at all open – confined to two or three 'black spots'. One of these is the C... Club, already decried by a moral welfare case worker:

"There is one other place, the C.... Club – girl after girl who comes here in trouble, says she met the man at the C... Club."

An investigator visited the C.... Club, and found it at first glance very quiet and well-behaved:

"The interior of the Public Hall in which the C... Club is situated seems excessively large for a meeting place for young people. Its size may in part explain the restrained behaviour of the youngsters present. Five minutes after opening time, an orderly queue of young boys was arrayed in front of the canteen. Most of the girls were seated on chairs down one side of the hall. In all there were about 70 boys and 30 girls present, age 16 to 23, mostly under 20. Of these only 2 boys were talking with girls ... the music started, girls danced with each other, boys remained by the canteen ... During the next half hour there was very little mixing between the sexes, it was very proper. In dancing, male partners held women always in the manner indicated by the text books, with no undue familiarity; bodies barely touching and male hands always in the place where they should be.
At 8.30 about twenty soldiers arrived in a bunch. They stood for a few minutes near the entrance, then some bought tea, others sat down and seven of them joined girls who looked as if they had been expecting them to arrive. From this point on the number of mixed pairs dancing increased. A few civilian males began to monitor particular

> *girls. At 9.15 there were 13 couples, all the rest remaining in groups of their own sex. No wandering hands, and there were no signs of covert love making."*

But towards the end of the club-evening, some couples left the hall for the dark, narrow side streets leading away [....]. The opportunity – if not the fact – of 'immorality' was quite clearly present. And an investigator's conversation with a club member suggested that some of the rumours about the Club had at least some foundation:

> *"Did you see that girl? She's a proper tart, she goes with all the soldiers – no, I don't think she gets paid for it. There's a bus with soldiers that comes half-way through the evening, she always gets one ... No, I haven't had her, but there's a few others you can get off with ... They aren't hard to get. It's all right if you buy them a cup of tea and dance with them a bit (Where you can go with them?) Oh, there's lots of passages round here, there's a passage just behind the Hall, you can always see one or two in there when the club shuts ...."*

An investigator verified with the proprietor of the semi-notorious common lodging house of the town that he would have no objection to a *"girl friend being brought in for the night"*. Town scandals were tracked down without much difficulty – but for the most part they seemed to be isolated incidents. Generally 'immorality', of a casual type at least, seems to be exceptional in Churchtown, and behaviour at public dances appears to remain at an exceptionally high level. The end of a dance at a Hall with a supposedly bad name, for instance:

> *"The dance finished at 10.30. Outside a number of women and girls waited on the pavement for friends. There was no conversation between the sexes, and no pick-ups. A couple who had arrived together and danced together all evening, came out of the hall, stood for half a minute talking, on the pavement, and then the man said "See you Saturday" and turned away. The girl called out an inaudible reply, turned in the opposite direction and walked quietly away alone ..."*

Observations at other dances told the same respectable story. Picking up was, to all intents and purposes, exceptional, and behaviour between acquaintances of the opposite sex seemed to leave nothing to be desired. Trying to probe deeper into this apparently high level of sexual morality, an investigator himself 'picked up' a girl at a Churchtown dance. Here are extracts from his report:

> *"A 25 year old working class girl seemed typical of the average girl at the Dance – and therefore a suitable victim for a 'picking up' exper-*

iment. She was fair and slim, rather washed-put looking, dressed in a simple 'Old Look' pale blue woollen frock. She danced in strict conformity with the local conventions – silent, technically efficient and at the end of the dance said 'Thank you very much' and went straight back to her girl friend. At the end of the second dance the investigator retained her in a one-sided conversation. She accepted a soft drink but seemed capable of little conversation. Returning to the dance floor, the investigator asked if he could take her home at the end of the dance... After a great deal of prevarication and hesitation, during the course of which she made it clear that Churchtown girls were different to the 'pretty fast' London girls, and after an unofficial investigation by her girl friend's boy friend, she at last agreed. At the end of the dance she and the investigator left together, and the following took place:

Investigator offered his arm to Mary, but she declined abruptly: "Oh, no."

Inv: "Why not?"

Mary: "You don't know what it's like here in Churchtown, it's not like London you know"

Inv: "I don't understand that"

Mary: "Well people talk here, you know.."

Inv: "What is there to talk about in a girl taking a fellow's arm while walking."

Mary: "Nothing really, but they do ... It would be back to my mother tomorrow. 'Who was that man Mary was with last night' that's what they'd say."

Inv: "What do they think if they see a boy or girl walking arm in arm?"

Mary: "Well they think they're courting"

Inv: "Does that mean that every time I see a boy or girl walking arm in arm I can take it for granted that they're courting...?"

Mary: "Mostly you can."

Mary said she had a boyfriend, and walked arm in arm with him. She conceded that she let him kiss her goodnight, but vehemently denied anything further:

Inv: "You don't mind him kissing and cuddling with you."

Mary: "We don't go in for that."

Inv: "You don't expect me to believe that, do you?"

Mary: "I don't care what you believe, it's true though"

Inv: "Are you trying to say that he doesn't try to make love to you"

Mary: "Oh, he kisses me sometimes, but I won't stand for anything else."

Inv: "Don't you ever go for walks in the meadows with him in summer?"

> Mary: "I DO NOT"
> Inv: "Where do you then?"
> Mary: "We go to the pictures"
> Inv: "And after the pictures?"
> Mary: "He takes me home ... I go straight indoors, we're not like the London girls you know"

All in all, allowing for a little reticence, this does seem to represent the pattern of contrasting behaviour and attitudes in Churchtown. A music hall comedian said, as part of his script:

> "Vice! Vice! They don't know what vice is here. That's what's the matter with Churchtown."

and, apart from its war memories, Churchtown's acquaintance with 'vice' does seem to be of the remotest kind. One of the few hints of any less respectable behaviour on a fairly wide scale came from a 28 year old working man who, having emphasised the difficulty involved in persuading a Churchtown girl even to be escorted home from a dance, conceded:

> "Oh, they're not all so chaste ... You can get a girl all right if you're prepared to start going out steady with them. I know for a fact that two mates of mine go through their girls regularly ... But they reckon it's all right, so long as they're going to get married."

Here again is the distinction between pre-marital relations between couples intending marriage, and sex relations of uncertain permanency – the former *to some extent* probably practised, the latter apparently generally rejected and frowned upon. But certainly morality at the verbal, conventional level sets very high standards; and equally certainly fear of social censure keeps outward behaviour in apparent conformity with the standards of respectability. Private behaviour – which in Churchtown is very private – is more difficult to assess, but we were not able to uncover much indication of any general deviation from the demands of conventional morality.

In Steeltown, the picture, official and especially unofficial, is rather different. Chapter 8 has already discussed the incidence of V.D. and prostitution in Steeltown; and it seems clear from this material that although the picture varies according to the angle from which it is viewed, the problem is considerably more serious here than it appeared in Churchtown. In a heavily industrial area with some bad slums as well as Dockyards, and with a visiting population of foreign seamen, the authorities are for the most part very much alive to the problem of prostitution and V.D. Even so, even in Steeltown prostitution seems to be largely confined to one or two relatively small and isolated parts of the town – particularly the Dock area. Generally, interviews with town officials show relatively little alarm. The National Officer of

Health for instance:

> *"I should say that, as a town, Steeltown is better than most other industrial towns. As a seaport, it is better than most. Standards of sex morality are far worse in such parts as Hull and Liverpool than they are here... we're not unduly worried about the incidence of VD cases, they have been remarkably static. I don't think we have a heavy incidence of it here, it's just that external factors have come along to increase the incidence. The main source of supply of disease in my opinion is the fact of foreign sailors coming into the town from the ships in the docks."*

The physician in charge of the town's V.D. Clinic, on the other hand, interpreted the same figures as 'very heavy'; compared with Churchtown situation they probably are. And looking at the matter from a quite different viewpoint, a Church of England Minister was equally pessimistic about Steeltown morality:

> *"There is a lot of immorality in towns, and I would say that Steeltown is fairly representative of an industrial town. You must remember that it is a port and there is inevitably a fairly flourishing 'Red Light' business ... Over by the docks and the railway there is a very low quarter; they have the lowest mental and moral standards. The housing conditions are such that children brought up there never know privacy, they are brought far too heavily against the hard facts of life from their earliest years ... As long as you have slums we shall continue to have a moral problem..."*

A Catholic priest insisted that *"Steeltown is not as black as places that are slightly larger."* And the Chief Probation Officer:

> *"There's nothing at all outstanding here as regards sexual morality. The prostitute problem is very small. It only affects a few... the police reckon dance halls and that are conducted in an orderly fashion, I think the standards of sex morality are quite high."*

The Chief Clerk to the Station Police Force told the same story:

> *"The standards of sex morality here are not bad for a sea port – It's all away from the public notice, in the docks and riverside, and in the market area where the loose women go drinking; but they confine themselves to these districts. Steeltown doesn't compare unfavourably with any other industrial town of its size..."*

The official picture seems clear. Steeltown is no better and no worse than any other town of its size – taking into account its docks and industries. More or less typical of a dock and industrial town, it seems fair to compare the unofficial picture with that of Churchtown – more middle-class, more rural, without docks, and much less industrialised. In Churchtown, it has already been seen, conventional standards are high, and fear of social censure exercises a strong inhibiting influence on behaviour which, so far as we could uncover it, maintains an almost equally high standard. Whether the unofficial picture of Steeltown...?

At night, Steeltown streets are noisier and more crowded than those of Churchtown. Couples can be seen in shop doorways or embracing in the streets, and the whole atmosphere is different. Railings are now put back round the park, but before this, according to the park keeper, the couples turned out at official closing time *"only waited till your back was turned to go back again"*, and sometimes stayed all night.

Churchtown dances are very quiet, and observation reveals almost no evidence of even the mildest love-making at them. At Steeltown dances behaviour is very different. Instead of the voluntary sex segregation that seemed to be typical in Churchtown, in a Steeltown evening the majority had paired off into couples, mostly dancing, some sitting down. Mild love-making goes on between a few of the sitting out couples. Social and sexual interest seems to supersede the almost exclusively technical interest in dancing apparent in Churchtown. Even the manner of dancing tends to be closer and more intimate, contrasting with the generally loose, impersonal textbook hold of Churchtown dances. Here is the picture towards the end of the evening at one of the more sophisticated dances, held a few miles out of Steeltown, but mainly attended by Steeltown people:

> *"During the later part of the evening – 10.30 to midnight – the chairs in one half-lighted recess are full, occupied almost entirely by couples, sitting closely together, arms round each other and cheek to cheek. Two couples, both under 20, have sat there for about an hour, the others for about half an hour or so, and then take their place.*
>
> *At 11.30 the floor is packed tight, people holding each other closely. About a dozen couples are sitting round the hall – four couples, all under 23 years of age, sitting on each others' lap, men's arms round girls' waists, and girls' arms round men's necks. Others are sitting in very close embrace, holding hands and men's arms round girls' shoulders and waists..."*

It is easy to understand the attraction that this dance hall has for young working class Steeltowners; there is drinking on the premises; it is held in a hotel; the band is first rate; the atmosphere is intimate and pseudo-night clubbish. The place is crowded out, and it is easy for a man to find a partner. If a reasonably presentable male wants to pick up a girl this is an ideal spot... The dance breaks up much later than at Churchtown functions:

> *"Dancers leave the hall at midnight, for buses back to Steeltown. At the end of the semi-dark corridor by the toilets three couples stand in corners, ages about 18, in each other's arms and kissing. On the way out, down the steps to the pavement, to the left and right in alcoves where there are seats, are about four young couples, arms round each others waists, kissing. On the pavement waiting for their buses, leaning or sitting on the low wall, are about 12 to 15 couples, various ages under 22, kissing, some leaning on each other, others sitting side by side. Other couples stand or lean, arms round each other's waists or holding hands...."*

A very different picture to the sober break-up of a Churchtown dance, where even walking arm in arm is frowned upon between couples who are not engaged. At the other Steeltown dances, on the other hand, the contrast is less striking. One of the twice-weekly Town Hall dances for instance:

> *"At 8.30 there were ten couples dancing, ages 17 to 25, 5 couples sitting out, 5 single girls and 15 single males sitting or standing out. A quarter of an hour later, 20 couples were on the floor, 18 dancing or holding each other in the conventional manner, two couples periodically changing their orthodox dancing steps to 'trucking' – walking side by side arms round each other. These two couples were holding each other tightly round the waist, looking into each others eyes, and talking softly ... At the end of a set of dances, only about a third of all couples walk off the floor together, holding hands or arms round each other's waist. The rest part company on the floor, and walk off singly ... Only one of the couples not dancing, who could be described as 'love making', are sitting on chairs next to each other, she with her hands resting lightly on his thigh, occasionally bending towards him and smiling into his face, he occasionally 'nuzzling' the back of her bare back or lightly caressing her bare right arm..."*
>
> *"By 10.15 the floor is quite crowded and the seats round the edge are practically full – about 60 people present in all. During the pauses between the sets of dances the vast majority stand in groups, pairs, or singly round the entrance door, the remainder sit on chairs round the floor..."*

This Steeltown dance breaks up in a more subdued way, but still differently to the Churchtown atmosphere:

> *"At 11.00 the 'King' and general exodus to the cloakroom. Five minutes later about 50 men waiting outside the cloakrooms, and another 30 or so waiting outside the Town Hall itself ... Men and women leaving all the time, the surprising majority of these leaving with members of their own sex, some saying 'goodnight' to ex-partners as they pass on the way out.*

Several working men standing at the top of the stairs leading to the exit. One 25 year old man to another 'What yer doing? – waiting to get yourself a woman?' The other – 'Bloody well got myself one – waiting for the bitch'. 'Ain't 'ave yer?' 'Yeh, but she don't come, don't expect she will – may have gone now. Might as bloody well wait and see'. Both go off after a few minutes, no woman having arrived.

18 year old girl to 19 year old, as they come out of the ladies' cloakroom, 'What a queue of men. Are they all waiting for girls, I wonder'. The other giggles, and they both hurry away arm in arm.

18 year old youth to 20 year old as he sees latter going down the stairs 'Waiting for a woman? They've all gone, you won't get one now'.

The crowd at the bottom of the stairs slowly disperse, the men mooning off in groups of their own sex, and girls coming out and walking off in pairs of two or three. Two boys would follow two girls for a few yards, call after them and whistle, but the boys would soon go off on their own. Only a minority of those coming out were in couples of opposite sex. Right at the end there were just about half a dozen youths, 17 to 20, hanging round the entrance to the Town Hall; then they too slowly moved off – some on their own, some in pairs..."

It is clear that in Steeltown expectations of picking up and pairing off by the end of the dance are higher than in Churchtown; and during the dancing itself, behaviour is much more openly provocative and sexual. This, of course, does not mean that immorality in the sense of extramarital sex relations or promiscuity is more frequent in Steeltown than in more inhibited Churchtown. This is suggested, on the other hand, by case histories collected by an investigator who had formerly lived and mixed in the town for two years in a personal capacity. Here, for instance, is the account of a 19 year old working class girl, given in confidence to that Investigator:

"I used to go out with another girl, we went to Bluebank, we always used to meet somebody to take to – just go into a coffee shop or somewhere and sit down, some chap would just come in and talk to you, ask you if you wanted another cup, or a cigarette and would sit down and there you are! They were soldiers or boys. Oh it didn't lead to love making. Might go to the pictures, or an amusement arcade, they would probably see us on the train, or come as far as Steeltown with us. We'd hardly ever get a compartment on our own, but when we did they'd kiss us and that; if we weren't on our own, they'd just put their arms around us. Nothing else when we were on our own in the compartment, that's as far as it used to go, just kiss of course and that's all. Sure, I wouldn't let them do anything else. Sometimes we'd make arrangements to see them again and go out again, to the pictures mostly. We only went to Bluebank on a Sunday – only day we could

see the soldiers – we never used to bother with anybody else – Don't know why – only sort of didn't.

I didn't like them that much for anything further than a kiss. I don't know about the other girl, she used to wander off on her own sometimes (with her boy).

She is now (two years later) married, she had to marry one of her boy friends as she was going to have a baby. She was consequently turned out of her home by her mother – nobody now knows where she went or what become of her.

These weren't the only boys we'd see – we saw others at the same time and they were mostly soldiers – we made arrangements to meet some of them the next Sunday, and then we'd meet some one else and go with them instead. It was only friendship – they just wanted a girl – You would meet a rotter – some of them would expect more from you – tried to be funny – you know – no need for me to tell you what they tried to do. They would shake with passion, I suppose it was, and their hands started to wander all over me – I'd tell them to get away ·and walk away and leave them.

I met Jack when he was twenty in the summer in the park [....]. I was introduced. I liked him. I saw a lot of him in the summertime in the park, and we went out occasionally together. I'd meet him at the Town Hall dance and he'd bring me home. He used to make love to me – real love – used to stand in the doorway – you can't make real love in the doorway – he used to try to do other things besides kiss and that. But I wouldn't let him.

Then one night I went to his house – about 8 weeks after I'd first met him. His mother and father were away on holidays – I think I knew they would be out – there were six of us – went to listen to some records.

The others went and I stayed. It just happened – we just sat on the settee, and he put his arms round me, then I lay on the settee – it just happened – I can't tell you how it happened. I didn't enjoy it – I didn't want to do it – I don't know why I done it, I must have been mad! I suppose he enjoyed it, he said he did. He seemed to whilst he was doing it.

Before this occasion I was a virgin, after that I realised I didn't like him at all.

I did go round again and his people were out, but it didn't happen again, I wouldn't let it happen – I refused. On that night he didn't use a contraceptive and my periods stopped. I knew what had happened. I took some stuff and skipped and skipped and skipped – had it given off somebody, eventually it was all right and my periods came back.

I've been out with boys but I've never felt anything for them until this next one, Ted, twenty four, in the merchant navy, whom I met twelve months later whilst staying at the hotel where I work. Later on he asked me to go out with him, went out on the Saturday night. He had supper at our house and took a taxi back to the hotel at 11.30 pm.

That was all right – just went on like that having a good time with him – He was a perfect gentleman to me for about three weeks. Ted always took me all over the place for dinner. He was a perfect gentleman. Christmas Eve, my day off and they were sailing any time. I went on the ship that day, he brought me off at midnight and 'taxied' me home – he sailed on Christmas morning. The first time he was here, after I've been out with him for about three weeks, he said 'lets go away from here for Christmas.' He booked a room somewhere in Newcastle, I believe, at a hotel.

We were going there for Christmas, but then we couldn't go as his ship was almost ready to go. He left on the Thursday and we were supposed to have gone away together on the Friday. I didn't think it was a very good idea, I was going because he wanted me to go. I don't think 'anything' would have happened – I don't really, he was perfectly all right the first twice he was here.

But it might have done once he got me away from here. About two months later he returned and he stayed again at the same hotel, I went out with him and it just happened, you know. When was the first time now? Well I don't know when the first time was.

It was in one of the hotel rooms. I went in and he invited me in. I can't remember the first time – I think I was drunk – no I wasn't – I was sober. It was a Friday – we'd been out all day, had lunch at my sister's, took my nephew to the park, had dinner in a restaurant and had two drinks – not drunk at all, came into the hotel at about 10 pm. and went into his room and it just happened. The lights were not switched on at all. I refused at first. He asked me and I said "Nothing doing", he said "Why not?".

I wouldn't have done it if I wasn't in love with him and he told me he was in love with me. I still love him though. I was sitting on the bed and he sat down beside me, he pushed me down on the bed, and put a pillow under my head, and he lay down beside me. I took my dress of, I would have got it very creased if I hadn't – nothing else. I didn't take a thing off except my shoes – I only had two more things on.

All the time I knew I shouldn't be doing it. He took most of his clothes off – and then it just happened. He used a contraceptive – I knew because I refused and he said it was quite safe – there was no danger – I agreed then. I didn't want to but I liked him and he wanted to. He said 'You can't be in love with me unless you will do it.'

We were there until about 2 pm.

It happened just once that night.

I don't know whether I enjoyed it or not.

I didn't enjoy it all because I was frightened, I would have done (enjoyed it) but I was frightened. I was in love with him. He enjoyed

*it because he told me he did. He said 'Didn't you enjoy it?' I said 'No,
I didn't because I was afraid.' He said he enjoyed it. I went off to my
room afterwards.*

(At this stage in the report she was trying to keep back tears from her eyes)

"*I don't know when it happened again – it happened twice more, in
the same place. Next time it happened I was drunk – We had a good
time and when we came in he was annoyed because I wouldn't consent to it again. He wouldn't speak to me the next day, but in the
evening he always spoke to me again, and at night time we'd go out
again.*

*Next time we went to his room and we went to bed – we stayed
there all night. I undressed, but not completely, I didn't want to. He
did undress properly and then it just happened – I suppose it happened several times through the night – about two or three times I
think it happened.*

*We didn't use a contraceptive, and I was awfully worried after-
wards. I was relieved of course when I did have my period afterwards.*

*I can remember I enjoyed it, he enjoyed it, he told me so – I think
that I enjoyed it. I was afraid even though I was drunk.*

*Then it happened again, a week ago tonight, I went to his room
again and it just happened. I told him I was worried, I was annoyed
with him. He said 'I don't know whether you'll be all right or not'. He
asked me what I'd do if I had a baby, I asked him what he would do,
he asked me when I should know if I was all right. I told him I should
be all right this Friday.*

*He said he'd see me if I was not all right. He said he loved me. He
thought I was 21, I told him I was.*

*Men want to be intimate without any understandings. I couldn't be
intimate with a man unless I was in love with him.*

*Men think you're terrible if you don't want to be intimate with
them – they want to know 'why not' and all that sort of thing.*

*He'd always give me my own way – very good to me, but he want-
ed something in return.*"

Our material suggests that this is no very unusual story for Steeltown – as far
any other largish industrial town for that matter. But it presents a very striking contrast to the Churchtown girl who would not even walk arm in arm, and
this contrast is typical of the different patterns of behaviour in the two towns.
What factors have produced such contrasting standards of morality? Quite
clearly industrialisation has been one factor in replacing the older conventions with a newer, less inhibited morality, but we can do little besides point
to the difference, without venturing too far into the complexities of the picture. What emerges most strongly from our material, however, is the fact that

morality is a [....] phenomena that is not one morality but many. Moral standards vary not only from one group to another, but also even within one group will be different on different occasions. Holidays, for instance, may turn morality upside down. In 1939 Mass-Observation surveyed sex behaviour in a Northern seaside resort, 'Seatown', the local holiday destination of another M-O study area, the industrial city of 'Worktown'. The war interval may have altered the facts of the material, but the holiday relation between the two places is unlikely to be much altered. Here is the Worktown sex picture, in so far as it could be publicly observed:

"In Worktown we must walk along the backstreets at night, after 11.15 when lights are all put out. There, at scattered intervals along the walls, will be closely-linked couples, standing, one or two in each back. Sexual intercourse enjoyed in this way (as common in winter as summer) is generally known as 'having a knee trembler'. It is the premarital or extra-marital method of all those Worktowners who have only the darkened back streets and who often cannot marry for simple economic reasons. It is easy to get a girl-friend in Worktown, if you can show yourself sensible, and have some money, and like cinemas or dancing or (less often) drinking. It takes some time to do anything you like with the girl, if it is possible at all – which it generally is. But this type of sex, backwall and knee-tremble, is only a fraction of the indoor married intercourse. In both there is a marked tendency to concentrate on the week-end, on Saturday night and Sunday early afternoon. The Saturday night out, at [a] cinema or central pub (see The Pub and the People) is partially preparation for this. Again, on Sunday afternoon when the children, whatever parental views, are sent out to Sunday School, you have time to 'forget about work', sex can be fully enjoyed, and intercourse is often downstairs on the sofa, called 'a soffey ender', such afternoon intercourse being termed a 'mattinay'.

The unemployed are widely supposed to have more intercourse more frequently, and our data indicates that this is true[,] as it is that they go to bed later, sleep longer. Shop assistants who have Thursday afternoon off often have their mattinays then. And if a chap wants 'a shot' during the week, O.K. 'if the wife is willing'. Decent men 'won't take advantage' of their wives, and this is a frequently-expressed point of view in Worktown's morals. Within this framework there is much sexual freedom, adultery, exchange of wives and 'living tally', though little promiscuity.

Bearing these points in mind, we may expect and understand a wide range of sexuality in Seatown, where a position parallel to that of unemployment is created. Certainly the Seatown backset is strongly sexual."

Whatever the degree of Seatown sexuality, the nature of sexual behaviour indulged in by its holdaymakers is quite different to the more primitive back-street opportunities which they enjoy at home in Worktown. In Seatown love-making is much more open and unashamed than in Worktown, and the picking-up rate is fast and continuous. Here, for instance, is the holiday diary of a mill-girl, again pre-war:

"Friday: Arrive at Seatown. Staying at Hull Road. Visit the tower, met 2 young men from Sheffield, went into the Bar and had a few drinks, afterwards dance, then on the promenade, strolled on the sands. Had supper at Cafe (chips and coffee) arrived back at digs 12 o'clock.

Saturday: Morning went a drive to Fleetwood, got back for 12.00 dinner.

Afternoon went to Pleasure Beach, picked up with 4 young men from Wakefield, had a good lot of amusement, enjoyed the Grand National best, went for a drink to the Huntsman. Evening went to the Tower dancing, from there to the Gardens and then back to the Tower, which we like best. Visit the Cafe garden for an ice. Listen to the Ladies Band which was playing the Blue Danube.

Sunday: Went to the Huntsman in the morning with four Scotch boys, stayed till dinner and then met them afterwards and went to the Pleasure Beach. Went a ride in a car to St. Anne's with four more boys. Arrived back at digs with boy friend 11.30.

Monday: Strolled on the prom with friends and met 4 Scotch boys, went dancing on the pier and drinks in the bar, enjoyed watching the Tight Rope Walkers and then went and had photo taken. Back to digs.

Tuesday: Went to the pier dancing, came off at 11.30 went up the Prom, went in Doctor Q, was very interesting show ... (No mention of being picked up Tuesday and Wednesday)

Thursday: Went to visit a friend, then had a stroll on the Pleasure Beach on my own, then on the prom. After tea went to the Tower dancing with the lady friend, came out, went home down the Prom, picked up with two young men from Preston.

Friday: Didn't go out while afternoon, went down to Pleasure Beach again on my own and then from there back up the prom. in the rain, it was throwing down and there was not a person to be seen.

Night went to Winter Gardens picked up with a sailor from New Zealand. Went and had a look round the amusement Id. machines, he won me two bracelets and a powder box. We danced and then home.

Saturday: Went with him to Pleasure Beach, and had a good round of amusements. He left at noon for Liverpool to catch his boat, I am leaving Seatown today."

Seatown evening shows such scenes as the following without restraint:

11.30 pm. for instance, a fine evening on the Prom:

> "The sea is rough, the sand covered.
> 2 men, 2 women. One of the girls lies on a form, knees pointing up, boy stands gazing down on her.
> 2 men walk slowly south, larger with left arm round other's neck.
> 1 man, 1 woman. Kiss, arms clasped round shoulders, 35 secs. Stop because girl gets on man's knees.
> 1 man, 1 woman, he fondles her breasts.
> 2 men, 2 women. Separate into couples. Kiss standing.
> 1 man, 1 woman. He gazes into her eyes. Kisses her neck, rubs her nose with his moustaches. They peck. She looks up. They talk. She clasps her handbag. They cuddle. She tries to press him to her lips. He kisses her neck. She rises from form, tightens her girdle. He presses her breast, drawing her down. They cuddle. He does not kiss her. They both get up, he towards the station.
> 2 men, 2 women. One man presses girl under him, on railings. Look at waves. Straighten to look at two people. Man eases position. Sticks out backside. Leaves girl, goes to left, blows nose and wipes mouth. Takes hanky out of right trouser pocket, puts it into left."

At 10.15 pm, of 82 groups on a strip of promenade, 54 were couples, 5 of those 50 were sitting down, 36 embracing, 8 loving, 9 kissing, 5 talking, 1 looking at the sea, 1 eating chips. From 11.30 to midnight, observation of 252 couples showed the following results:

Sitting down and embracing..120
Standing and embracing. 42
Lying on sand embracing 46
Sitting kissing 25
Necking in cars...9
Standing kissing 3
Girl sitting on man's knees. 7

Moreover these couples lack the incentive of privacy. The report continues:

> "For older men of scoptophilic tendencies as well as barracking young men, the sands at night are a happy hunting-ground. Whenever a couple gets down on the sands, they very quickly have a ring of silent, staring, immobile individuals round them. This is particularly the case in the dark shadows of the Central Pier. Apparently immune from rebuke verbal or physical, silent circles surround each couple, observing their manoeuvres from a range of less than two yards."

The Seatown illegitimacy rates for 1936 was the highest in England for that year, and represents one to every 1,900 of the resident population. Statistically, there was a 9 to one chance of every woman having an illegitimate child. But it is significant that examination of illegitimacy figures according to season showed that the holiday-makers themselves had no notable effect on local high rate of conception for this year. Only in so far as he diagnoses Seatown home life – with a consequent observation of round-the-year morals – and imbues [the] resident morality with something of the holiday-lifting of summer sanctions, can the Worktown holiday maker be saddled with the responsibility for Seatown's record illegitimacy rate.

But it is clear that holiday standards are very different to the morality of all the year round. Picking up is more often and more constantly 'the thing'; love making and 'immorality' may not be more frequent but it is certainly less secret, more flamboyant and unashamed. The annual holiday may produce sexual behaviour attitudes that the rest of the working year could scarcely recognise.

Chapter Eleven: Opinion Forming: Vanguards and Resistance Forces

Whichever direction opinion is moving in, it is not without conflicts and skirmishes constantly on the way. It is important, therefore, to see how people have lined themselves up for battle – to discover who is on whose side.

On the whole opinion on sexual topics seems to be moulded chiefly by two major influences – education and religion, each pulling in broadly opposite directions. Generally, the higher people's educational and social grading, the more tolerant they appear; church-going, on the other hand, is more liable to accompany a relatively rigid moral outlook.

Educational level, social class and income, are all too closely interwoven with each other not to pull in roughly the same directions. People with the higher social gradings are most inclined to accept the principles of birth control, divorce, and sex education and they also more often condone extra-marital relations.

Acceptance of birth control also increases strikingly with income – but on this issue at least, educational level seems to have much less influence. Birth control is approved by:

41% of those earning less than £3 a week
65% ———- " — up to   £10 a week
71% ———- " — over   £10 a week

Poorer people use birth control less than the financially better off, perhaps partly because of the financial cost of contraceptives. But very few people make any direct reference to economic factors such as this, and lower income disapproval is more likely to derive from vague and inadequate knowledge. It seems more likely that poverty operates in a more direct manner in producing disapproval of divorce. Here again the money aspect seldom comes explicitly into attitudes, but probably only the better-off regard divorce as any sort of practical possibility for themselves; for people in the lower income groups divorce can safely remain morally out of bounds whilst it is beyond their personal reach.

Illogically, members of the higher income and educational groups tend to see not only divorce but also marriage in a more than usually wholeheartedly favourable light; but this is probably because the better off less often come up against the material inconveniences of marriage than those who often lived in cramped conditions or are forced to provide for a large family on a small income. Perhaps another result of similar background, the feeling that sex is indispensable to happiness tends to increase with social grading – even though education and social class are also inclined to make people more susceptible to the suggestion that there may be potential dangers attached to sex. Better-off people focus particularly on the fear of 'overdoing' sex relations, and are also especially inclined to rule out relations that seem to be affectionless or in any way abnormal.

Not only in attitudes to birth control, but also in the way people look at divorce, whether or not people go to church is less important than the effect of the type of church that they go to. Roman Catholics, of course, are more consistently hostile to divorce than any other group we were able to study. Opposed to divorce were:

69% of all Roman Catholic church-goers
29% of all Church of England church-goers
29% of all Non-Conformist church-goers
27% of all Church of Scotland church-goers

It is on these two main issues that the effect of religion emerges most strikingly. Non-church goers are a little the more likely to condone prostitution and extramarital relations and to qualify their approval of marriage with cautious reservations. On the other hand they are also more inclined to accept the principal of sex education, to feel that sex is indispensable to happiness and to resist the idea that it may be in any way wrong. If there is an 'emancipated' outlook on sex, it belongs to the non-church goer.

Other group differences of outlook are less striking and less consistent. Age wields an influence over attitudes chiefly in producing a pessimistic assessment of current moral standards amongst older people, as well as an increasing wariness of the possible dangers of sex; older people, particularly, are inclined to stress V.D. and 'overdoing' sex relations as a source of potential harm to the husband. They are less willing than younger people to approve of sex education or birth control. But on the evidence of age influences alone it would be tendentious to forecast any change in sexual behaviour.

Social surveys that cover most general topics usually show a tendency for women to show less interest than men, to have fewer ideas and to cling to the more conservative and socially acceptable type of opinion. On sexual topics, however, this usual result emerged less clearly. Women were quite as interested as men in the questions that were asked them, and they equally often had an opinion to offer. They were even more willing than men to accept the comparatively new principle of sex education. Only when people were asked about prostitution and extra-marital relations did the old standard pattern reappear: one man in four accepts or condones extra-marital relations, and only one woman in every seven; again, one man in four accepts prostitution, compared with one woman in ten. More strikingly, women are far more inclined than men to feel that happiness is possible without sex – but they also less often suspect it of hidden dangers. Men, understandably, are more wary of contracting V.D. and they are also more inclined to dwell on the consequences of over-frequent sex relations.

Finally, there are indications that political Leftishness also has some influence in effecting sexual freethinking, but this factor was on the whole left uninvestigated by our present survey. The effect of class and education seems slightly stronger than the influence of church-going, and as education becomes more widespread it is possible that the sexual tolerances that go with it will also gain in frequency; at the moment there is in England only slight evidence of even minor increases in church-going. Nevertheless, church-going and religious belief are closely related to people's outlook on sexual topics, particularly to those on which the Church itself has officially most to say. But on the whole the issue of sexual freedom and tolerance reduces itself to a conflict between the older traditions of the official Church outlook and the 'freethinking' endeavours of the more educated middle and upper class.

Appendices

Appendix One: The Sex Habits of a Group

Throughout this report there are scattered references to the sex habits of [the Mass-Observation] National Panel of Voluntary Observers. This chapter sets out to co-ordinate these references, to bring them together and expand them into a rounded picture of the sex habits of a single relatively homogeneous group.

[....] [The] M-0 Panel [....] is by no means representative of the population at large. Self-selected both through its capacity for introspection and its interest in sociology as well as self-expression (its members sit down once a month to write lengthy expositions of their views and habits on specified subjects), it is on average less reticent than most people, as well as more than usually intelligent and well-educated. In addition, the fact that [....] [a proportion] of the present Panel group originally joined Mass Observation in response to an appeal in 'The Statesman and Nation' means that the group as a whole is disproportionately Left in politics and outlook. Looking at them in this light, it is important to discover just how far their opinions on sexual topics diverge from those of the population as a whole:

91% of the Panel approved of sex education
67% of the street sample approved of sex education

53% of the Panel approve unreservedly of marriage
58% of the street sample approve   "   "   "

79% of the Panel approve of birth control
63% of the street sample approve "   "

63% of the Panel more or less approve of divorce
57% of the street sample more or less " "   "

24% of the Panel are against extra-marital relations (note 1)
63% of the Street sample " "   "   "

51% of the Panel are against prostitution (note 1)
60% of the street sample "   "   "   "

It is clear that the Panel group is more in favour of sexual freedom than the street sample. This difference is in line with difference within the street sample, which shows that sexual 'progressiveness' tends to increase as people's education level rises and their religious orthodoxy declines. It is also likely that approval of sexual freedom is more widespread amongst the politically Leftish. But if the attitudes of Panel members show an above average favouring of freedom, the same might be expected to be true of their habits; certainly there are some slight indications that the tendency to indulge in pre- and extra-marital adventures increases with income. On the other hand, it is possible that the situation in England is similar to that explored in America by Kinsey. In that case the Panel group, at its relatively high educational level, will only be [slightly] more inclined than the street sample to indulge in the sexual outlets of homosexuality, masturbation and petting to climax (note 2) – and actually less inclined to have premarital sex relations or intercourse with prostitutes. In these two latter ways (ways, moreover, in which 'immorality' is commonly conceived) the American equivalents to our Panel group are more 'moral' than the rest of the community.

Sending out *attitude* questionnaires to our National Panel of 1,000 members, we received 642 replies – roughly our usual return. 600 of these agreed to fill in a second, personal questionnaire on their sex *habits* and 450 sent this back completed. This gave us, in all, a 25% loss on our usual rate of return; quite clearly this lays open the possibility of an additional source of errors in our results – since the 25% who either refused to receive the questionnaire or else failed to return it may represent selected portions of the Panel group. Certainly there were some who felt that their sexual life was so quiet and normal as to be unworthy of description, and others (unmarried) who failed to reply on the grounds that they had no sexual life at all. On the other hand, many may have been ashamed of the range and unorthodoxy of their sexual outlet. Reticence can have divergent causes, which we can only hope have cancelled each other out; we have at least no grounds for supposing a higher proportion of replies on this subject are from exhibitionists and cranks than we normally receive on any question.

Finally, before presenting the results, there is the question of internal validity. Naturally, all the information that has been given us may not be entirely honest. People may be suppressing facts about themselves where they feel them to be shameful, or, on the other hand, they may boastfully exaggerate them. We have no objective way of checking on either of these two tendencies, but *so far as is possible to judge* neither is very pronounced. Only very occasionally did we feel that replies were deliberately exaggerated: indications of the reverse trend occurred more frequently. Sometimes, for instance, a respondent would confess to great difficulty in admitting some aspect of his sex life; when asked whether there was any part of the questionnaire that particularly embarrassed them, nearly half mentioned at least one part, usually their erotic day-dream and masturbatory habits, particularly the latter. Compared with the frequency with which it is practised, homosexuality, too, was relatively often a source of embarrassment. But apart from this there is little evidence of people being seriously embarrassed or ashamed by the questions they had to answer; on the subject of sex relations outside marriage particularly, there is no evidence at all that replies have been softened down in the direction of conventionality. Nevertheless, it is best to regard the following summary of results as an approximate estimate of the actual picture – doubtfully exaggerated, more probably to some extent toned down.

The Unmarried

About one person in five claimed to have had no love relationship of any kind with a member of the opposite sex. A further quarter of the unmarried were engaged to be married, or else had been at some time in the past; a quarter had a 'particular friend of the opposite sex' at the time of answering the questionnaire, and the remainder had enjoyed at least one such relationship in the past.

Physical experience of love-making from a member of the opposite sex is, however, rather more extensive; only about one in every seven said they had never known love-making in even its mildest form. This draws at least a margin of people who must have experienced only casual love-making of a more or less purely physical kind. Men admit to a greater desire for physical intimacy; only one unmarried men in ten claimed that he had never wished for sexual intercourse, compared with one unmarried woman in every three.

Physical relationships – with or without a background of affection – are more frequent amongst single men than single women, although emotional relationships are about equally common for both. Among these single people:

92% of the men had experienced some love-making, compared with 72% of the women
70% of the men had experienced intimate love-making (note 3), compared with 51% of the women
49% of the men had had sexual intercourse, compared with 38% of the women

Not only do men more often admit to physical desire and experience, but they also apparently find it easier to get satisfaction from these relationships; in both intercourse and intimate love-making, they emerge as more capable than women of achieving a physical climax, and even in pre-marital affairs most say they usually experience one. But for men and women alike, sexual intercourse tends to become more satisfying with marriage. Only one unmarried person in ten described the relationships he had experienced as generally (not necessarily climactically) satisfactory; the most common reasons for dissatisfaction are, in the order in which they are most often mentioned:

physical discomfort and fear of interruption
lack of ardour on the part of the woman
lack of affection between the two
aesthetic or other objections to contraceptives used
moral conflict

Asked in [a] direct fashion about contraceptives, about half of this unmarried group said that they interfered with their pleasure; most used a sheath. Faith in the safety of contraceptives, moreover, increases with marriage. With these doubts about contraceptives in their minds, it is not difficult to understand why unmarried sex relations apparently involve so high a rate of dissatisfaction.

In the extent of pre-marital intercourse, the present habits of the unmarried group conform closely to the pre-marriage habits of the married. Roughly two in every five of either group say they have had pre-marital experience. Almost all of those who are now married and have ever experienced pre-marital relations have done so, with or without further experience, with their present husband or wife. And of the married people without experience of pre-marital relations, nine-tenths of the men and two-thirds of the women say they would have liked it. Moral objections seem to have provided the most frequent deterrent; only one person in every sex mentioned a restraining fear of pregnancy.

Amongst married people, pre-marital experience with someone other than the present husband or wife is much less common; about half the men reported this type of experience and only a quarter of the women. Many of the men said that they had experienced intercourse before marriage with a wide variety of partners – one in seven of the married men had had pre-marital intercourse with more than four women, and in the majority of cases they were not in love with these pre-marital partners.

Those who had desired this sort of sex relations but held back gave the following reasons, each mentioned by about one in ten:

fear of pregnancy   ) mentioned about equally by
moral objections   ) men and women alike.

shyness   ) mentioned
lack of opportunity) almost exclusively
fear of V.D.   ) by men

Finally, after marriage, these who have had pre-marital experience are apparently neither more nor less happy than those who have done without it.

Marriage

Three quarters of the married members of this group said that they were satisfied, often very satisfied, with their married lives generally; proportions were identical for both men and women. Only about one in twenty was definitely unsatisfied. Answers, such as this one from a thirty-year old husband, come frequently from both young and old:

"I am very satisfied. I have been very clever or very lucky in my choice of partner."

Contentment with the purely physical aspects of marriage is about equally frequent. Nearly three-quarters say they are satisfied, physically as well as emotionally. But in this case the difference between the sexes is very marked, 82% of the men saying that intercourse with their wives leaves them completely satisfied, whilst only 61% of the women are satisfied after intercourse with their husbands. Only three in every five of the women of this group experience an orgasm as a result of intercourse. Out of every hundred women:

18   always experienced a sexual climax
42   nearly always experienced a sexual climax
11   sometimes experienced a sexual climax
21   never or rarely experienced a sexual climax
8   gave miscellaneous replies – that they 'used to' or failed to before having a child

There is a very marked relationship between this ability to feel satisfied after intercourse, and general satisfaction with marriage. 87% of the happily married (men and women together) are satisfied after intercourse, but only 42% of the unhappy. 17% of the unhappily married seldom or never feel satisfied and 13%, though physically sated, feel no emotional pleasure.

Easier male satisfaction in intercourse also emerges from discussion of what, if anything, would make for a more satisfactory marital relationship; four men and only three women in every ten said no improvement was necessary. The improvement most often desired was that the sexual partner should be physically more co-operative and passionate during lovemaking; this was mentioned by about one person in seven – and almost as often by women as by men. The improvement next most often mentioned was that the husband or wife should be a better lover emotionally – but this is mainly a woman's grievance, mentioned by one woman in five and one man in thirty. Women tend to complain that their husbands are emotionally unsatisfying and allow them too little preliminary lovemaking and endearment. Here are some typical comments:

> "My husband accused me of being 'cold' but little knew the passion-
> ate longing I experienced. I only he had made love to me instead of
> using me like a chamber pot" (middle aged woman)

> "If my husband had ever said a word of love or endearment or
> thanks" (50 year old woman)

> "Apart from a kiss and a cuddle we have no intimate love making.
> I've tried to tell him but he's so clumsy (I think through shyness) and
> I'd rather be left alone" (37 year old woman)

The only other major reason for dissatisfaction, mentioned by more than one
in ten, is the necessity for birth control. But this is more often an unmarried
complaint. Men usually complain on this score because of the mechanical
difficulty; women because they wish they could have more children.

Notes

1 Since many people mention special exonerating circumstances in their replies, it
is simpler for purposes of comparison to consider merely those who are against
prostitution and extra-marital relations.
[2 This is one of the very few mentions in the text of 'Little Kinsey' of heterosexual sex which is not 'intercourse'; see also note 3 below.]
[3 This was defined in the questionnaire as *"love-making which stopped short only
of intercourse"* [....]. The questionnaires themselves contain a good many mentions of sexual behaviour in addition to intercourse.]

Appendix Two: Homosexual Groups (note 1)

Throughout this survey, Mass-Observation concentrated on attitudes to the normal rather than the abnormal. But quite apart from the difficulty of defining what is normal or abnormal behaviour, it is impossible completely to separate the two in any discussion of sex. Our questions provoked constant references to abnormalities of one kind or another – usually left very vague – and it is clear that fear of indulging in something that it is believed other people do not do constitutes an important source of restraint. A good deal of dissatisfaction and anxiety could be removed if more people knew more about the wide range of sexual behaviour.

Variations in the frequency of sexual relations emerge as the source of much uncertainty and self-doubt. Apart from evidence that has already been given, one in [....] of the M-O National Panel regards himself as abnormal in as much as he is 'oversexed', and another [....] feels that he is under-sexed. But in addition to the question of frequencies, and still coming within the bounds of heterosexual relations, are variations of kind; [....]% of the M-O Panel admit that sado-masochistic elements come into their erotic fantasies and 2% of the married members of this group feel that their sex relations with their wives could be improved by the inclusion of sadistic or masochistic variations.

[....] One in five of [the] M-O Panel have experienced homosexual relations of one degree or another. Investigating a national sample of American men, Kinsey found that as many as [....] had experienced some physical form of homosexual behaviour [....].

There is no doubt but that homosexuality in one form or another is at least not an unusual form of sexual behaviour. Yet popular feeling against it is very strong. It was Mass-Observation's original intention to include a question on homosexuality in the present survey (with the result that the pilot questionnaires produced a limited amount of material on this subject), but difficulties of time and finance meant that this had to be excluded from the final questionnaire. Results of the pilot surveys, however, suggested that about a third just did not understand what homosexuality (note 2) was, *"it never occurred to me"*. About a quarter just represented themselves as generally against it, and another third showed very violent reactions, calling homosexuality *'disgusting'*, *'terrible'* and *'revolting'*:

> *"I think that's terrible. Really, I can't describe it, it makes me feel embarrassed to be near anyone like that"*. (28 year old wife of newsagent).

> *"I think it a terrible thing – absolutely detestable"*. (41 year old storekeeper).

> *"It's a bit of a teaser. I shouldn't think they're human – it is done, I know – I mean animals don't do that, I shouldn't think."* (48 year old coal depot manager)

Another reaction, less revolted, was the *"rather vulgar, isn't it?"* from a 6 years' married carpenter. A few people, on the other hand, look at the matter from a more or less clinical angle and suggest some form of treatment. A sales manager:

> *"That is an abnormality that most people regard with horror – but it is a disease of the mind that could be given treatment."*

But on the whole people regard homosexuality as a revolting or incomprehensible form of behaviour; many would even seem just not to have heard of it. It is, of course, impossible to generalise from such limited results as these; but the isolationist manner in which homosexual groups appear to function makes extensive ignorance of their existence at least a possibility. Mass-Observation was incidentally able to collect a small amount of observational material on homosexual cliques. The exclusive nature of the group, with its distinctive outlook, isolationist activities and chance of making contacts, can be judged from the following extracts from one report. The chief members of this group are Arthur, a young musician, John, a receptionist, Michael, a secretary, and Peter, a clerk.

Homosexuality (note 3) 6.7.49

[A. Arthur, 25, a young musician and a homosexual, first introduced investigator to other homosexuals.
B. John, 30, receptionist in a large London hotel.
C. Michael, 28, private secretary to a prominent public figure.
D. Peter, 19, clerk in the film industry.]

John and Michael have been living together for about eight years, for the last eighteen months in a town centre flat. In the early part of the war, Michael saw John's phone no. in the house of a homosexual friend; later that evening whilst fire-watching and having nothing to do he remembered this phone no. and dialled it, introduced himself and the conversation lasted for an hour and a half. Five conversations followed [during] the next five days, at the end of which time they met, liked each other very much, and within a few weeks were living together.

These two only move in 'queer' circles – they are not at all keen on the company of non-homosexuals except for neuters, borderline cases and possible converts. All queers are welcomed by John and Michael and hospitality heaped upon them.

One year ago Peter was picked up in Piccadilly by Michael after having been followed for 20 mins. – "Hullo my name is Michael what's yours?", Michael said as he caught up with Peter. They spent the evening together drinking and talking. Peter was taken to Michael's flat and they slept together, Peter being passive (as he is to this day) and Michael active (as essentially he is). A month or so later John met Paul, a French youth of exceptional physical beauty who now stays with John several times a week in the flat.

Paul has now returned to France and probably Peter will return home to Ireland within the year (Peter is in love with Michael but realises that it is unrequited and he is only a temporary bed partner). In which case John and Michael will return to their twin beds and their conjugal life together.

Peter is now living on his own in the flat and has a prostitute from the next flat to prepare his meals and look after him.

Arthur recently saw an advertisement in a London evening paper to the effect that a 'Disciplinarian' was willing to pay holiday expenses in France for a suitable male companion. Arthur recognised the word Disciplinarian as being the trade name for a sadistic homosexual and as Arthur is essentially a masochist (plus many complex variations) he answered the advertisement. It turned out that Charles – the advertiser – wanted somebody who he could love (he believed he could love Arthur) and who would in their turn completely and utterly subordinate their self to Charles. Somebody who would willingly submit to Charles' sadistic desires.

Charles wanted Arthur alone with him in a bedroom dressed only in a special pair of very tight short pants and was then to allow Charles to wield a cane on him as much and as violently as Charles deemed necessary. After caning Charles was prepared to satisfy any sexual desires Arthur might have, i.e. masturbation, fellatio, redicato etc.

Arthur was in raptures over the prospect of such a holiday with Charles and was completely prepared to take his role in this flagellative partnership. He told inv. that Charles was beautifully developed and that they would get on very well together.

Michael is a completely unabashed individual, very polished in his behaviour and manners, quite at home and strong in any company. Seems to have adopted an almost Wildean attitude, in conversation never at a loss for a witty retort or an apt remark – usually with a suggestion of sarcasm or sneering. Queers' conversation thrives on ambiguities of a sexual nature i.e. intentionally misinterpreting a harmless remark to be suggestively sexual (homosexual).

Fairly frequently, John and Michael have held soirees at their flat – for queers only, at which unknown queers (e.g. inv.) are introduced and weighed up. At these soirees behaviour is usually quite reserved, things seldom progressing beyond the point of a caress of buttocks (Peter has most prominent protruding buttocks which are continually being caressed and slapped by Michael) or thigh, holding hands or kissing (quite apart from the promiscuous kissing of arrivals & departures).

It is at the parties solely and strictly reserved for known queers that more advanced love making takes place.

On Easter Sunday, Arthur, Michael, Peter, inv. and Frank (a rich young man of 35 with a car – a recent addition to this group) went to Brighton by Frank's car. Frank is the clandestine type of homosexual and essentially an active type. He heartily disapproves of all varieties of 'camp' (i.e. flaunting the fact that one is a queer, see below in the pub) and, unless he was known as such, would never be identified as a homosexual, except perhaps by being in the company of a more overt type of homosexual.

Peter wore white shirt & flannels and sandals. Arthur, Michael and inv. white shirts, shorts (rolled high to expose as much thigh as possible) and sandals. Michael had a powdered face, and powdered hair tightly curled which he would continually pat into place and curl on his fingertips.

A third of the journey was spent in serious discussion – cars, music & plays. The rest of the time was spent in discussing boys and youths on the road, walking, cycling or motoring: "My God! just look at those legs – perfect." , "What a divine physique, & what thighs.". Or sometimes there were just deep-down sighs and long full expressions. They were in fact the reactions comparable to those displayed by heterosexual males completely lacking in inhibitions, when seeing beautiful girls scantily dressed.

Lunch was eaten on the cliff tops, east of Rottingdean, after which photographs were taken – subjects posing so as to expose as much of their legs and in the most photogenic manner. Toes to the ground and the pelvic girdle slipped to one side....

Early evening was spent in strolling up and down the promenade in the vicinity of the 'Men only' beach – which is a notorious haunt of homosexuals – and from which several were observed to leave. This strutting along the prom in white sandals, rolled up shorts, white short sleeved shirts and sunglasses was a suggestively 'camp' action and objected to by F. who nevertheless accompanied the others.

Michael and Peter walked along the prom. from Hove to Brighton where they would meet the rest, they would not say why they were going off on their own. Arthur assured inv. that they were going with the sole intention of seeing who they could pick-up or flirt with.

An hour later all met by the Palace pier and it was decided to spend the rest of the evening in a pub. Michael knew of several places where 'queers' congregate....

Arthur, Michael, Peter & inv. went into a small bar which was completely full of about 35 males – the vast majority of whom appeared to be homosexuals. All those that subsequently entered were recognised by inv. as being queers. About half a dozen present were recognised by C. as being a 'notorious bitch' or a 'perfect sod'.

Four others in two pairs were introduced to the group as old friends of Arthur and Michael – who had come to Brighton from London for the day. Both these pairs inv. later discovered were 'married' and living together. Another queer was recognised by Arthur and introduced to the group – he was a resident of Brighton and working in London.

Michael was rather carried away by the environment in this 'queers' bar and was given to draping himself over the staircase railings, smiling around the room, speaking loudly and exaggerated gestures and mannerisms. Peter got more and more annoyed at [Michael,] eventually accused him of being 'camp' and walked out in a temper, Michael then being somewhat 'put out'....

Notes

[1 This Appendix is the most unfinished of the draft edited chapters and is in a clearly different form from the others. The first section is typed and hand-edited in Len England's handwriting. The second section is handwritten and edited in another hand, by 'GP'.]

[2 Defined in the question as 'sex relations between two people of the same sex'. It must again be emphasised that this question was only included in the preliminary piloting of the survey.]

[3 The original handwritten second section, before it was edited, presumably by Len England or 'GP', is more explicit about the sexual goings-on between this group of men.]

The Feminist Surveys Back

Chapter 6

Surveying the Survey

'The Feminist Surveys Back' and 'Surveying the Survey' are titles that invoke the earlier social science meaning for the term 'survey', that of providing an overview, a focused and analytically scrutinising gaze. It was in this sense that Terence Young, involved in one of the Mass-Observation shopping surveys and on the fringes of the 'Economics of Everyday Life' project, produced a detailed, but neither numerical nor statistical, investigation of the conditions of social life in the then-new housing areas of Becontree and Dagenham for the Becontree Social Survey Committee[1]. The Becontree Social Survey Committee and the funder of this research, the Pilgrim Trust, thereby supported a non-numerical and non-statistical overview produced from the centre of the British 'survey movement'. Alan Wells, providing a contemporary 1936 guide to the different kinds of concerns and emphases within this movement, includes this older sense of 'surveying' as an important aspect of it and sees it as by no means antithetical to the newer components[2].

In the 1930s fetishism of the number had not yet come to mark 'the survey' and to provide the dominant meaning of the term in a social science context. At this time the social sciences were considerably more fluidly related to each other than we are accustomed to now, in the 1990s. Certainly the boundaries between the social sciences, regarding not only substantive focus but also and perhaps more importantly methodological procedurals[3], were in the process of being reworked and made both more obviously present and more consequential in terms of professional status, publications and career paths. However, there were important contrary developments. There was, for instance, the cross-disciplinary response to the challenge of Mass-Observation represented by the methodologically-focused collection edited by Frederick Bartlett and others, *The Study of Society*[4]. This collective response is indicative of longer-standing collaborative intellectual links between the social science disciplines that provide a frame within which other contemporary cross-disciplinary activities can be located, such as a series of 1930s conferences concerned with the role of social science within what was seen as a likely expansion of higher education. Closely related to this was the concerted effort on the part of a number of important social scientists of the day, Philip Sargant Florence and John Maynard Keynes among them, to ensure that a 'synthetic social science' would be at the heart of this probable expansion in the form of economic sociology[5]. Such developments were linked to, in some measure were a response to, the growing fragmentation of 1930s social science, as new approaches and ideas and theories came into existence alongside the old. Not only was sociology, perhaps unsurprisingly, a composite of a number of such divergent emphases and approaches, so too were the apparently more 'scientific' and unitary disciplines of economics, psychology, anthropology. It is in this context that the considerable success of calls for a synthetic 'economic sociology' must be placed, attracting some of the key figures from across all these discipline areas.

Through the 1930s, 'surveying' was both a methodological development located within fragmentation and diversity, and was itself composed by fragmentations and diversities: thus surveying as a general overview rubbed shoulders with census-like surveys of total populations, with the use of experimental and control groups, with the development of ideas about random sampling. Present-day commentators[6] usefully have noted that there were commonalities here, that the variants within the 1930s survey movement had several unifying characteristics: they proceeded from fieldwork, the first-hand collection of data, to provide a comprehensive coverage of an area or locality; they analysed social units (individuals, families, households) and not just aggregates; and these developments were closely related to ideas about reform and changes in public policy. However, all three factors also characterize much, perhaps even most, of Mass-Observation's research, including that which was least 'survey'-like in its approach; and the first two are almost defining characteristics of the anthropological and sociological development of ethnography as a fieldwork method over the same period of time that saw the development of 'the survey'. It would seem, then, that such commonalities were even more common, characterizing new developments across different disciplines and methodologies, and were by no means confined to the survey as such.

The 1939–1945 war saw major changes here, heralding and promoting the development of 'the survey' into its current dominant form, along with two related factors. The first was the development of theoretical ideas and methodological practices connected with random sampling, and the second was the use of mechanical and computerized methods of data analysis. These related developments had enormous post-war reverberations in sociology, for the research events of the war had indicated that sociology as a discipline might find a place in the funding sun through government support of a 'big science' policy-oriented forms of social research. Mass-Observation in fact played a role within this. A number of its research personnel went into the Government Wartime Social Survey, and one of these, Geoffrey Thomas, became the Director of the Government Social Survey after the war. Later Mass-Observation crossed methodological swords with British Institute of

Public Opinion (BIPO) about market research methods in relation to random quota sampling methods, occasioning Mark Abrams' critique of Mass-Observation's allegedly 'slipshod' approach[7]. Closely related here is the sea-change constituted by 'Little Kinsey' its rapid methodological move from an observational and 'characteristic' Mass-Observation study to a random sample survey. As my discussion below argues, one of the most interesting things about 'Little Kinsey' is that the resultant survey data were then placed within a very different epistemological and analytical frame that under-cut and decentered the generalizing impulse of the survey and prioritized the explication of difference within the sample. Later still, after the 1949 organizational changes that occurred around the design, conduct and analysis of 'Little Kinsey', Mass-Observation Ltd gradually conformed to the canons of standard market research practice; the text of 'Little Kinsey', produced on the cusp of the change, bears the hallmarks of both 'phases' in the life of this complex and fascinating organization.

My own 'survey' in Section Three takes two forms. First, as a feminist I 'survey' in the older sense of an overview, by looking in detail at the structure, content and arguments of 'Little Kinsey', Second, I provide an overview of 'the feminist surveying back', looking at the work of a particular feminist who surveys in the more specific present-day meaning of the term, in the form of the sex surveys of American researcher Shere Hite. It is particularly appropriate to discuss the work of Shere Hite here, not only because hers is the most considerable and sustained feminist attempt to map, and from this to theorize, 'the sexual' and its relationship to social change, but more especially because the methodological form of Hite's particular variant on 'the survey' brings her surprisingly close to the methodological form adopted in 'Little Kinsey'. The sex survey work of Hite, like that of 'Little Kinsey', seeks to combine a representative breadth of coverage with something considerably harder to achieve: a prescient grasp of the pulse beneath, indicators of the meaning of behaviour and also of what people do with their experientially located knowledge of the sexual and its complex inter-relationships with the social. 'Little Kinsey' and the work of Shere Hite have similar methodological and epistemological sources and are thus interestingly 'compared and contrasted', as examination papers often phrase it.

Notes

1 Terence Young (1934) *Becontree and Dagenham*.
2 Alan Wells (1936) 'Social surveys and sociology'.
3 See here Morgan and Stanley (1993), pp.1–25.
4 Bartlett *et al.* (1939).
5 These matters are discussed in detail in Stanley (1990a). See also Adolf Lowe's (1935) *Economics and Society* for perhaps the most important intellectual expression of the 'synthetic' approach.
6 See for example Marsh (1982a, 1982b); Bulmer (1982a); and Bulmer, Bales and Sklar (1991) pp.2-4.

7   However, as argued by Summerfield (1992) with regard to its wartime research, Mass-Observation swiftly achieved results that, with hindsight, were incredibly accurate; this was in spite of – indeed I would argue more strongly it was because of – its eschewing of 'strict' sampling and survey procedures. The debate was about the form that market research should take, with BIPO and Abrams standing for an emergent and rapidly canonical 'science' in survey methods and procedures, and particularly with regard to sampling.

Chapter 7

Surveying Sex the Mass-Observation Way

'Little Kinsey': Textual Voices and Rhetorical Facts

The research that became central to 'Little Kinsey' is composed by three related surveys. The first is a 'street sample' survey of over 2000 people selected by random sampling methods carried out in a wide cross-section of cities, towns and villages in Britain. The second is a postal survey of about 1000 each of three groups of 'opinion leaders': clergymen, teachers and doctors. The third is formed by the results of a 'directive' (a set of interrelated questions written in a Mass-Observation house style) and a follow-up directive sent to members of Mass-Observation's National Panel, with responses from around 450 members. These related surveys are reported upon in tabular form (usually in whole percentage terms – 'out of every hundred, X responded....'), at a number of points within the text. These numerical statements are embedded in an extended argument developed around the topic on which each chapter focuses, and they are surrounded by extensive quotations that were written verbatim by the interviewers as they worked through the questionnaire with members of the 'street sample'.

Cross-cutting the quantitative and the qualitative material from the three surveys is an earlier Mass-Observation textual 'voice'. This is formed by extensive quotation from reports, by Mass-Observation researchers who had worked in the 'Churchtown' and 'Steeltown' phase of the research (in the chapters dealing with prostitution and sexual morality in particular); by Mass-Observation researchers who had worked during the late 1930s in 'Seatown' (Blackpool) in a considerably earlier project (there is a long quotation from this in the chapter concerned with sexual morality); and by a Mass-Observation investigator who wrote about his research on/involvement in a 'homosexual group'. This 'voice' constitutes different kinds of rhetorical strategies within the text, and its presence has the effect of subordinating the 'quantitative' to the 'qualitative'. However, the dominant rhetorical strategy is that of the Mass-Observation analyst/writer of the text. This was Len England, a man with a long-term involvement in Mass-Observation, and then later in Mass-Observation Ltd[1].

Three competing rhetorical strategies exist in 'Little Kinsey', which in a sense speak past each other about different kinds of data and 'facts' about sexual 'habit' and opinion, and they are articulated using: first, quantitative data from the three surveys; second, qualitative data collected alongside the street survey; and third, observational reports from other Mass-Observation projects. Surrounding these is an argumentative structure that articulates these others in a fourth strategy, that of the *sotto voce* analyst/writer himself, apparently absent, without gender or class, without a 'point of view'. This textual complexity and diversity constitutes what is almost a signature for Mass-Observation writing over the period 1937–1949, a signature that signs away a single authoritative authorial identity in favour of a polyphonous and multi-layered set of textual 'voices' or strategies, which, by their very diversity, signal that no one of these is to be seen as *'the* voice'. There is 'authority', but at the same time authority is rhetorically dispersed.

This dispersal of authorial authority is given additional emphasis by the way that the survey data is used. Only infrequently are categorical conclusions drawn about 'people and sex', for the methodological treatment given to 'the numbers' interrogates these around multiplicities of difference: through comparisons of differences between the three different survey groups; and through statements of differences within each survey group by age, education, income, sex, by whether people lived in villages, towns or cities, and whether they were church-goers or not. The result is that almost every statement of 'this' has alongside it an alternative one concerning 'that', with both being presented as 'fact' and 'true' for different groups and individuals.

Read this way, 'Little Kinsey' can be seen as a memorial to the failures of data triangulation[2]. This is triangulation seen as strangulation, the mass of resultant data choking away the ability to state 'the facts' with any clarity. Almost every piece of numerical analysis is used to produce a multiplicity of 'ends', a fracturing of categorical statement that represents actual variability within the population. However, a concern with untidy 'ends' of data, that is, small and apparently 'insignificant' groups of numbers, is something that contemporary survey practice has turned its face away from in favour of the categorical, the analysis and representation of dominant trends and research clarity. Such a 'scientific' denial of untidy life to produce neat research does not appear in 'Little Kinsey', and its 'failure' in this regard constitutes an extremely interesting attempt to grapple with the very real complexities involved in investigating the social and sexual.

'Little Kinsey', therefore, can be read in another equally plausible way, as an epistemological murder rather than a methodological suicide, as the murder of 'the facts' and any notion that these 'speak for themselves'. Interestingly, the text of 'Little Kinsey' at one point states that the facts must be allowed to do precisely this, speak for themselves, but then, ironically, throughout it provides *alternative* facts, depending on social location: on people's class, age, sex, religious affiliation, locality, and whether they were surveyed, interviewed or observed. The movement of Mass-Observation, from being an organization concerned with methodological eclecticism within an observational framework focusing on actual behaviour, to becoming a market-research organization concerned with surveying and tabulating attitudes, was not achieved without difficulty. The text of 'Little Kinsey' is testimony to this, for it demonstrates the epistemological divide between the two approaches and that these different data actually construct different phenomena, which in the final analysis are irreconcilable. The fact that 'Little Kinsey' was not published contemporaneously is closely related to this: its analyst/writer was unable to achieve a form for the text that achieved closure over the different kinds of data, and, relatedly, such closure and hence authority was increasingly seen as necessary, not only by Mass-Observation's researchers but also by the wider research community in Britain.

Theorizing Sex the Mass-Observation Way

'Little Kinsey' theorizes, albeit in a largely implicit way, sex, or rather sexual conduct (that is, not only behaviour, but also emotions, thoughts, feelings, imaginings); and it does so around elaborative contrasts built up from an initial distinction between sexual 'habit', Mass-Observation's term for repeated behaviour, and sexual attitudes. These interconnected contrastive themes have a wider remit than 'sex' conceived narrowly, for they provide a guide to understanding social life, social structure and social action more widely.

'Little Kinsey' starts with the Preface and Tom Harrisson's comparison with the Kinsey study of sex and the human male. On one level the Preface rejects the notion that 'Little Kinsey' is in any sense an appropriate title, emphasizing that Kinsey's research involved considerably larger numbers and employed a more resolutely statistical stance. However – and perhaps typically so for Harrisson – there is considerable irony here, for overtly rejecting the name 'Little Kinsey' actually brings this title, catchy and easily memorable, to public attention and associating it with this research. The Preface is equally double-edged in drawing distance between Mass-Observation's research and that of Kinsey, emphasizing that it is both less and more than Kinsey's and making a virtue of both – the 'less' is a virtue because there are fewer tables and 'science' and, relatedly, the 'more' is also a virtue because there is more of the 'actuality' of 'the real life' provided by Mass-Observation's approach. By the latter the Preface is refering to the extensive use of interview and observational material, insisting that no known method can produce total accuracy and that those which approach this tend to lose the 'human' element by distancing themselves from what real people do in all its complexity. It is clear, then, that 'less science', in the form of fewer tables and numbers, is desirable because this enables more 'real life' to appear.

The main text continues this approach, in particular through the distinction introduced in the first few chapters between 'habit' or behaviour and attitude. This distinction is seen to involve the relationship between truth and experience, with experience and behaviour being that which gives the 'true picture'. This brings what is ostensibly a report of survey data about attitudes, produced at the cusp of the change to the market research-oriented Mass-Observation Ltd, perhaps surprisingly close to Mass-Observation's earlier insistence that direct observation provides the only proper data about social life. 'Little Kinsey' strongly argues that, the nearer to people's own lives, the more they will speak from experience instead of using 'other people' as their reference point. 'Attitude' is thus seen to exist when experience is lacking, and to be largely the views of 'opinion leaders' of different kinds. Stripped of 'Little Kinsey's random samples and tables, this critical stance towards 'attitude' could easily have appeared in the very earliest Mass-Observation writing, from about 1937, in which Mass-Observation insisted on direct observation of behaviour (including talk recorded verbatim by its investigators), in contrast with the then-emergent and social psychology-influenced market research obsession with attitude.

'Little Kinsey' discerns a 'faint unease' about sex among its sample members, an ambivalent movement between sexual desire and fear, especially by women, who are described as finding sex more distasteful than men. 'Little Kinsey' notes people's considerably greater ease in being questioned about sex, women as much as men, than had been expected. However, it interprets women's frequent articulation of dislike, distaste and boredom with (hetero)sex and their resentment of men's patronage of prostitutes and involvement in other extra-marital sex as 'sexual conservatism'. This results in a textual inability to 'hear' what a good many women, and some men, actually say. Thus, that women are more in favour of early sex education than men is explained away as women 'really' wanting this because of telling girls about menstruation. Similarly women's fear of unwanted pregnancy is seen as 'really' a fear of sex, and women's anger about prostitution is recast as 'really' envy and jealousy. Indeed when men are quoted expressing similar views, this is treated in exactly the same way, as the product of outdated conservatism. Such an essentialist stance, seeing 'sex' as a 'drive', an inner and determined impulse that propels social and sexual behaviour, was becoming fairly common through the conjunction of popularized Freudian ideas with those of social *avant guardism*: if 'they' think sex is bad, then 'we' think it good; if 'they' think it should be peripheral, then 'we' think it must be central; 'they' do not want social and economic change, and 'we' do. The effect is to deny, by explaining away as 'really' something else, the commonsensical constructionist approach taken to 'sex' that characterizes a good deal of quoted responses, presenting this as an 'anti-sex' conservatism rather than the understanding that sex could and should be different and better.

This contrast between sexual conservatism and sexual progressivism is continued, for (moral) approval and disapproval of sex, particularly in relation to sex education, is discussed in 'Little Kinsey' around a number of sets of overlaying contrasts. One of these is between the 'educated' and the 'church-going', with what is 'progressive' being associated with the former and what is 'conservative' with the latter, and with women characterized as more conservative and morally censorious than men in spite of their promotion of earlier sex education. A more general – and stereotypically Freudian – approach to sexual progressivism and sexual conscrvatism is then developed through attempting to correlate the sex 'habits' of sample members with three aspects of parenting: whether their mothers were 'clean and tidy'; their parents' sex attitudes; and whether they experienced conflict with their parents. Although no statistical correlation of adult behaviour with these childhood factors exists, the text proposes that negative statistical results can still mean that significant relationships may exist, because the statistical can mask and hide the behavioural – indeed, this argumentative thread about statistics masking life runs throughout the text.

This is a wider argument than the sexual, for the text associates the 'progressive' more generally with whatever is most 'pro-sex' (an attitude of course not unknown amongst self-styled sexual vanguards today), and this in turn leads to the dismissal, denial or ignoring of any questioning of the assumption that sex is *the* centrally important feature of human life. Such questioning comes predominantly but not exclusively from women, who reject the idea that sex (i.e. sexual happiness) is necessary for happiness more generally. This is an important point, for it belies the emphasis in much later sex research that sex is so important that sexual unhappiness or dissatisfaction will necessarily affect the totality of a relationship and a life, a point that I return to later. People's questioning and rejection is not least of the essentialist and masculinist assumption that this means only 'sex (*for men*)' which appears in what many male sample members express and also, although more ambivalently, in the stance taken by the analyst/writer.

The assumption of heterosexuality in 'Little Kinsey', along with the associated assumption that 'sex' is synonymous with penetration, occurs less through overt statement, more through the weight of the content of the successive chapters on the 'facts of life', sex education and birth control. Each of these associates 'sex' with 'where babies come from'. The street sample questionnaires certainly included questions on non-penetrative behaviours, but little of this beyond one brief mention appears within the text of 'Little Kinsey'. (Hetero) sexuality appears as predominantly a male phenomenon, and one which is also a 'drive' and thus the determined product of 'nature'. It is consequent on this that the necessity of sex outside marriage is conceded, because 'men are human'; while prostitution is seen to be 'demand-led' by men's sexual 'needs' rather than 'supply-led' by women's economic necessity and is condoned because of 'masculine *human nature*'[3]. However, there remains an ambivalence, a hint and perhaps more than a hint of irony in an accompanying statement about the '*uncontrollable male*'. Still, the overall implication is that 'sex'/heterosexuality is more a male affair, not least because discussions of the street sample are frequently invoked through the phrase 'the man in the street', through references to what the male part of the sample said, while 'the woman in the street' simply vanishes.

Sexual knowledge and sexual ignorance is most fully discussed in relation to the role of language around the example of 'birth control', with the text conjecturing whether the low level of response here demonstrates a problem of terminology or a problem of ignorance on the part of sample members. This occurs around what is described as sample members' 'confusion' of birth control with controls over the birth process, and also with abstention and coitus interruptus, rather than with what the writer sees as its 'proper' meaning of a variety of (mechanical and chemical) contraceptives. This raises a wider issue, noted by the sex surveys after 'Little Kinsey', concerning the language used in sex research, when neither formal nor 'everyday' terms may be appropriate or even familiar to many if not most people, for sexual behaviour may be typically not spoken about at all, even within long-term marital and sexual relationships.

The relationship between necessity and morality is seen in 'Little Kinsey' as the source of the clash that the writer discerns between habit (behaviour) and attitude (opinion) in people's responses to the survey questions, for attitude and morality are seen to cohere when people react, not from experience, but instead by reference to what they suppose they *should* think because they assign such a view to 'important' people. Thus, moral disapproval of birth control is treated textually as not 'rational', merely as being the 'ruling idea', an interpretation that is also applied to people's ideas about spacing childbirth and also divorce. However, the difference between necessity and morality here, and its perceived relationship to behaviour and attitude, is a considerably wider one within the framework of 'Little Kinsey'. Experience is seen to have signal importance in the production of knowledge, for 'Little Kinsey's' stance is that the nearer something is to their own lives, then the more likely people are to speak from direct experience rather than through invoking what 'other people' supposedly think. The contrast here is with social attitudes, relied upon when people do not have first-hand knowledge and produced in a stereotypical way. This perceived gulf between the knowledge formed from experience and the stereotypes formed around 'attitudes' is indeed pursued through much of the substantive discussion in 'Little Kinsey', regarding unhappy parents, marriage and divorce, prostitution and other kinds of extra-marital sexual relations.

What is invoked by 'Little Kinsey' as 'natural' is crucial to the perceived relationship between sex, marriage and children: 'sex' is that which produces babies, and it is this that constitutes 'the facts of life' which are the subject of sex education and birth control and are the substance of what marriage is all about. However, the perceived 'naturalness' of what is 'normal' is also seen to be both socially constructed *and* to have limits: the un/naturalness of sex occurs around the boundaries set by its nature and its frequency. Sex as biologically constituted and 'natural' occurs within marriage and produces children. However, sample members suggest that 'natural sex' can become 'unnatural' where there is sublimation and repression: if taken 'too far' in some unspecified way, perhaps by being engaged in outside of specifically procreative sex, it can become uncontrollable and so unnatural. Similarly, the frequency of sexual behaviour is seen to traverse the boundaries between the natural and unnatural; and again notions of the possible uncontrollability of unfettered sexual habit are referred to here.

At various key junctures, women's patent dissatisfaction with 'sex' is expressed in the text. In one woman's graphic phrase, she had been 'used as a chamber pot' by a husband who, in terms of 'habit' at least, divorced sex and emotion and saw 'sex' as an entirely penetrational act. These dissatisfactions are so clearly articulated to today's ear, accustomed by successive researches and public discussion and debate of sexual behaviours and trends, that it seems almost incredible that their presence in the text can be treated as almost transparent by the analyst/writer of 'Little Kinsey'. And yet, there such statements of women's longing, boredom, distaste, certainly are in the text; and, just as certainly, there they are 'unheard'. So how to explain this?

One way to explain it is to draw a temporal (and gendered) distance, and say the time had not yet arrived when such statements could be 'heard' and understood, at least by a male author. However, there is another and in my view more plausible explanation, drawing on the 1945-published Mass-Observation research on Britain's falling birth-rate, which centred women's dissatisfactions and their refusal to live lives like their mothers' and which related sexual changes to changes in perceptions of relationships and in the changing social and economic possibilities – that is, to a wider pattern of dissatisfaction that encompassed the sexual but which was not determined by this.

The different rhetorical strategies outlined earlier are crucial to understanding the successes and failures of 'Little Kinsey'. In Mass-Observation's *Britain and Her Birth-Rate*[4] a textual closure had operated because the entirety of the research had been concerned with representing one point of view, women's. Here marriage and child-birth (and, presumptively, (hetero)sex) were seen from a single textual viewpoint, that of the women who were giving birth to fewer children more widely spaced. 'Little Kinsey's' writer/analyst had a considerably more difficult task: how textually to represent a multiplicity of different and competing 'voices', only one of which is that of 'the women', speaking anger, sadness, rarely complete satisfaction, while representing these within a framework that has abandoned the 'female-as-norm' stance of *Britain and Her Birth-Rate* for one that is written in apparently ungendered terms but which actually accepts the 'male-as-norm'. This analytic failure is not that of the writer/analyst in any simple or personal sense; it is rather something that derives from the theorization of 'sex' which underpins 'Little Kinsey', the textual acceptance that 'sex' (penetrational, done by men to women) is normative and innate and so natural as to be effectively unquestionable. The problem for the analyst/writer was thus how to satisfactorily represent difference, the difference and questioning of women, while also writing from an almost unquestionable 'male' point of view. It is by no means surprising that 'Little Kinsey's' author could not solve what was, in this formulation, unsolvable; what is of enormous interest is that he came so close to succeeding, to fully representing difference, complexity, fragmentation, within a coherent textual strategy.

'Little Kinsey' includes but does not 'hear' the voice of those women who said that sexually and emotionally they were disappointed, alienated and bored and that they wanted a good many things to change, principally men and their (sexual and other) behaviour. This failure is importantly connected with the theorization of 'sex' that underpins and informs the structure, content and interpretation of this research. 'Little Kinsey' is premised upon the innateness of heterosexuality and its synonymity with 'sex' itself because the 'facts of life' are those of penetrational heterosexuality, or rather of men in penetrational mode, and, from this starting point, 'Little Kinsey's' subsequent discussion of sex education, birth control and marriage follows. At various junctions, however, this set of assumptions is cross-cut by other data from the research. At a number of points, the lack of fit between the frequency with which both homosexuality and masturbation occur, and the surprised outrage of people's 'attitudes' to these behaviours, is noted in the text. In addition, there are two further and perhaps more significant challenges to the presumed innate naturalness of 'sex'. The first is people's frequently expressed distaste for the narrowly penetrational and 'animal' form that (hetero)sex takes, expressed by men as well as women, although more women are quoted to this effect. Perhaps paradoxically, the second derives from the almost ubiquitous assumption of the 'naturalness' of sex. As the text notes, for most people the 'naturalness' of sex is both socially constructed and has interactional limits, for what is 'natural' can stop being so by virtue of the frequency of its occurence or by the specific nature of variants within it; and of course both 'variants' and '(over)frequency' depend upon the acceptance of normative standards that are presumptively conformed to by 'other people'. The normality and naturalness of penetrational heterosexuality is then perceived as normatively inviolate, but in behaviour practice shaky and dependent on normative judgements of self against other and, considerably more seditiously with regard to women, of experience against expectation.

Such an understanding of the contrasts between the normative and the behavioural is closely related to what 'Little Kinsey' takes as a crucial distinction between attitude and habit, opinion and behaviour, morality and necessity, ignorance and experience. The role of experience in the production of (first-hand) knowledge is central here, for 'Little Kinsey' throughout distinguishes between behaviour and experience, which enable people to 'speak for themselves', and the articulation of attitudes, which are seen as frequently misguided or simply incorrect. It is perhaps no accident that 'Little Kinsey' at various points notes women's tendency to speak from what they are directly involved in, indeed to provide statements expressed through examples, with men giving voice to general attitudes not experientially located in this way.

From this it might be expected that, rather than not 'hearing' what women were saying about their sexual and emotional involvements with men, 'Little Kinsey' would be fully alive to women's dissatisfactions. Certainly the text contains many articulations of this, but what is absent is the recognition that it constituted a motor force for change that so startlingly marks Mass-Observation's research on Britain's falling birth-rate. 'Little Kinsey' certainly notes that sexual change has occurred and is still occurring, but what it does not 'hear', and so cannot bring together analytically, is the importance of women's *general* dissatisfaction with the kind of life that their mothers led, and how this might connect with their *specific* sexual and emotional dissatisfactions. Both are present in the text, but hostages to the role assigned to 'progressive' views about sex, which lead the writer to assign women's dissatisfactions to sexual conservatism against the assumed norm of men's sexual progressiveness. 'Little Kinsey's' central rhetorical positioning of a 'male-as-the-norm' stance derives from its implicit theorization of sex as not only normative but also causative; and it is this which prevents it from analytically coming to grips with the very sources of change it had set out to investigate.

However, in my view 'Little Kinsey' moved considerably further in the direction of explaining wider social change and its links to changes in sexual and marital relationships and experiences than the other British sex surveys discussed in this book, including the National Survey. Its methodological approach, and the resultant competing rhetorical strategies or 'voices' that characterize the text of 'Little Kinsey', which represented failure for its writer/analyst and contributed to its non-publication, is what makes it insightful and challenging by enabling it to show the diversity and complexity of people's lives, attitudes and behaviour.[5] Moreover, its methodological approach has more in common with that of Kinsey than Tom Harrisson's Preface allows,[6] and these commonalities bring both surprisingly close to the methodological approach taken by feminist sex researcher Shere Hite, whose work also assumes the causative centrality of the sexual and sees women's desire for social and economic change as stemming from sexual dissatisfactions.

Notes

1 As discussed with Len England in a personal interview, Len England/Liz Stanley, 22 August 1990. The manuscript report on 'Little Kinsey' was written over 45 years ago, and Len England did not recollect the details of its writing.

2 That is, the use of three different kinds of data generated by different methods: ethnographic, interview and survey data, for instance. The implicit assumption is that these data simply provide three different 'angles' on the same social phenomenon, whereas an epistemologically more informed view on data

triangulation insists that these data are ultimately unreconcilable because the perspectival or epistemological frame within which each is located actually constructs the 'same' social phenomenon differently.

3 p. 208, original emphasis; herein seen pp. 152–3.
4 Mass-Observation (1945), *Britain and Her Birth-Rate*.
5 I have focused my discussion on methodological and epistemological issues; the details of method, in the narrower sense of technique, are discussed in detail in Stanley (1995).
6 And perhaps more than Harrisson knew about, given the then paucity of detailed published information on Kinsey's research process and interviewing style; see here Weinberg (1976).

Chapter 8

Shere Hite and the Feminist Sex Survey

Hite's work has interesting, indeed intriguing, similarities to and differences from 'Little Kinsey'. Her work is of course by no means alone in providing a feminist view on sex and sexuality, and nor is it alone in researching sexual behaviour either. Feminist analysis of the sexual is both plentiful and spans different approaches and emphases, and it includes interesting theoretical ideas about sex and sexuality as well as practical investigations of sexual behaviour[1]. My concern, however, is not to provide a broad overview of the range of feminist work concerned with sex. My concern, as I explained in the Introduction, is with the *sex survey*, not sexual theory, nor sex research conducted through interviews or other kinds of qualitative approach. Indeed, my concern is not with any kind of survey, but specifically those based on national random samples and thus carried out in the framework of 'big science'.

The 'big science' form of the survey has achieved a particular kind of canonical status. Its respectability in research terms is closely related to assumptions about the generalizability of its results to the general population; and its popular status derives from the belief that the 'findings' of an academically and scientifically respectable survey are 'the truth' and therefore indisputable. My approach is instead that such findings should be seen as the products of a particular way of 'seeing', a particular way of investigating and interpreting the social world and making knowledge-claims about it, claims which are as disputable as any other 'point of view' and any other way of investigating and interpreting social life[2]. My criticisms are particularly directed at the privileged status of 'big science', a status that I can discern no good epistemological grounds for granting. This is not to say that I do not find the survey an interesting and useful, although limited, method; and nor is it to say that I do not find its post-war achievement of canonical status and epistemological privilege quite fascinating. It is important to take seriously the emergence of the scientific importance assigned to the survey in an analytically informed way, and my examination of the post-war 'career' of the British sex survey should be seen in this context. A part of my professional and sociological career has been as a 'survey researcher', outside as well as inside of academia[3]; my comments are appreciative although critical, but certainly not dismissive; however, they are also the comments of someone who is not 'a believer'.

I use the term 'believer' to characterize those who do not see, or rather who do not accept, that there are *fundamental* problems – political, or ethical, or methodological, or epistemological – to an approach. In this sense I am a non-believer in *all* social science methods, discerning at least some such problems with them all. However, such a methodological agnosticism is not shared by the majority of social scientists, nor perhaps by the majority of feminist social scientists. Many, perhaps even most, feminists in the social sciences have placed themselves on one side or another of a divide between the quantitative ('hard', scientific, and for some also masculine and thus objectionable) and the qualitative ('soft', radical, feminist if not feminine, and so acceptable). Such a binary way of thinking about methods in gendered terms I regard as far too simplistic, for it removes by fiat the epistemological, and also the ethical and political, difficulties that are to be found with every 'method', every form of social investigation, including those like interviewing which have achieved almost canonical status within feminist social science[4]. In my view, feminist attention should instead be directed to social inquiry at the level of epistemology, for it is the epistemological frame that methods and their data-products are located within that condition the knowledge-claims that are made from them, and therefore their likely wider political and social impact[5].

There are, however, many feminist social scientists who to one degree or another align themselves with foundationalism, or the survey method, or both. There are those who are 'believers' in this approach, those who see it as intellectually or practically preferable in spite of its limitations, those who want to make political use of the fact that other people are 'believers', and there are those who make the transition from one of these other positions to 'believing'[6]. It is important to take seriously their arguments about why they find the survey approach a, more or less, satisfactory one to work within, why they feel able to position themselves epistemologically in this way. My particular interest has been engaged by those feminists who make the same kind of epistemologically-based objections to the (contemporary) survey approach as I have done, but nonetheless who continue to seek good, sensible and feminist ways of re-writing its most basic assumptions and procedures and products. The work of Shere Hite is important here, as the most popularly visible feminist proponent of the sex survey approach, and I now go on to consider some of these wider arguments through looking at her research.

Thus far I have focused on the developing sex survey tradition largely within one national context, that of Britain, although recognizing the importance of Kinsey's work in stimulating its development. National contexts provide an intellectual and an organizational frame that importantly and consequentially affects: what can or can not be said; how it can be said; who the audience will be; the relationship between researchers and policy-makers, and between the survey and other kinds of social science; and popular opinion of what these different kinds of investigations mean. Therefore, I look at the work of Hite, then, as I have done with Kinsey: in spite of its American origins and because of the interesting equivalencies between her work and that of 'Little Kinsey'.

The published accounts of Shere Hite's substantive research each bear the title of a 'report' – *The Hite Report on Female Sexuality*, *The Hite Report on Male Sexuality*, *The Hite Report on Women and Love*. They thereby make direct reference to the Kinsey reports on male and female sexual behaviour, although in a way that also signals a distance from these for fairly similar reasons to those provided by Tom Harrisson's Preface to 'Little Kinsey' – their lack of the 'real stuff' of human sexuality, its emotions, feelings, thoughts and meanings as these reverberate within people's lives and behaviours. The substantive content of Hite's research has proved every bit as controversial as its methodological approach, not I think because this is particularly new, but because it has been articulated by – shock, horror – a feminist and in such a very high profile way as to capture media headlines, something that has occurred not least because Hite has chosen to work using surveys with very large samples, using 'big science' but in ways which considerably depart from some of its central precepts.

The aim of Shere Hite's research has been to 'define or discover the physical nature of [women's] sexuality'[7], exploring the full range of women's sexual experience and sexual response so as to find out what is common and therefore physiologically-based. Hite's central means has been through a questionnaire that has gone through a number of successive changes and developments over the period of her research, starting in the early 1970s as 57 detailed questions to which respondents could provide written answers to all, or some, or by combining questions. One version of this was provided as a 'fold out' back cover to her first book, *Sexual Honesty*, which published some of the replies to the earliest form of the questionnaire. By the 1987 publication of *The Hite Report on Women and Love*, this had increased to 127 questions.

The first of Hite's books to present her substantive findings was the 1976 *Hite Report on Female Sexuality*. This sees masturbation as the sexual baseline, and notes that, in spite of women's supposed 'orgasmic dysfunction', the vast majority of women easily and quickly experience orgasm from masturbation, and do so with an intensity of pleasure they rarely experience in orgasmic sexual acts with a partner. Most women, this Report argues, do not experience orgasm during heterosexual intercourse, which is initiated, controlled and ended by men, while women enjoy it to the extent they do because for them it signifies the greatest intimacy that men can provide. Most of the minority who do have orgasms during intercourse do so because they ensure that what are, for them orgasm-producing behaviours are part of this. The majority of women who do not have orgasm during intercourse tend to see this as 'their fault' and to withdraw emotionally as well as sexually. This

Report notes that men see this as women being less 'liberated', or as not 'needing' sex as much as them, and argues that most men have little insight that a combination of their unsatisfactorily limited notion of 'sex' as specifi-cally penetrational, combined with an incapacitating inability to express emo-tional intimacy in any other way, alienates women. Most divorces, it points out, are initiated by women, and women who divorce often prefer dire pover-ty to the continuation of their marriages. The so-called 'sexual revolution', the Report emphasizes, is propelled by men moving from one failed rela-tionship to another, with women feeling that more effective contraception has removed the possibility of refusing sex 'legitimately'. Women, it argues, have not yet had a sexual revolution and are in search of a real one, for many are tired of the 'male sexual pattern' and men's emotional incapacities dominat-ing their emotional and sexual lives; and many of those relationships with men that do last do so because these women spend a good deal of time and energy changing men's behaviours.

This first Hite Report conceptualizes sex less as innate or determined, and more the product of a set of choices conditioned by social expectation, knowledge of the possibilities, and habit: choices that many women are com-ing to re-think and re-make. It proposes that masturbation for many women forms the basis of their most intense sexual pleasures; a good many women from early adulthood on define their sexuality as either lesbian or bisexual; while other women recognize that their most fulfilling emotional relationships are with women friends rather than male sexual partners. The continuing attachment to unsatisfactory men is construed, in part, as women's condi-tioned need for men's acceptance and good opinion, in part economic depen-dency and intimidation: the *sexual* politics of heterosexuality.

The 1981 *Hite Report on Male Sexuality* focuses on what men think, and feel about sex, whether this is changing, and how emotions relate to the rest of their lives. The emphasis is on what has been neglected in previous work: women's orgasms in the first Report, men's emotions in the second. The ana-lytic concern continues the theme of change: whether there are differences between cultural convention about 'sex' and men's own sexual feelings, what sex as they experience it means to them, and whether this might provide the groundwork for redefining their relationships with women or with other men. Many men, this Report proposes, are dissatisfied and unhappy; but they are unable to effect any real change because they are caught in a convention that gives them power and control and defines 'sex' for everyone around the mechanics of what will give men ejaculation in the shortest time. In relation-ships with women they become angry and resentful at women's emotional demands on them at the same time that women withdraw from them sexual-ly, but most cannot do without women's emotional energy and support. Many men see 'sex' in its narrow penetrational sense as what 'a man' is; most believe that men *should* initiate, control and terminate sex and that anything else is outside the realms of the conceivable. They resent any attempt by women to move away from such a narrow notion of 'sex', seeing this as women's lack of sexual liberatedness compared with them, coupled with their widespread repulsion regarding any closer encounter with women's genitals. With regard to emotionality, most men cannot understand the fuss that women make, seeing 'sex' as a sufficient expression of emotion, and thinking they are doing their best by wanting 'sex' but being then unaccountably rejected for this.

The 1987 *Hite Report on Women and Love* continues this analytic move from sex and orgasm to emotion and relationships, following the ideas and arguments expressed by respondents. Its main concern is to document '*a great change women are making in their lives*', for over 98% of the women respondents '*say they want to make basic changes in their relationships and marriages, improve the emotional relationships they have with men*'.[8] Most men do not, apparently cannot, talk about their feelings. The majority of women experience this as men's emotional withholding coupled with a fear men express as resentment of emotion in others, which stems from equating intimacy with loss and weakness and consequently with 'being like a woman'. Men are perceived, thereby, as deliberately maintaining power and control in relationships; the emotional contract in heterosexual relationships is that women give emotions, men take them, a structural non-reciprocity.

The consequence is that many women have changed their ideas about not only sexual relationships but their lives in general. In practice love is not the centre of their lives because men have not allowed it to be, and this is increasingly fuelling other changes, other life choices. Women's dissatisfactions have led to what Hite presents as a historical turning point,[9] the detailed discussion of which is headed 'To transform the culture with our values'.[10] Here the theme of contemporary social change and women's part in it is explored: 'women's dissatisfaction: driving social change', 'women... the driving force behind change'.[11] Men cannot, or will not, change because this would make them more like women, she argues, and being like a woman is something most men despise as weakness, and they fear it would lead to them being rejected by other men, something more fundamentally important to them than being rejected by women. The vast majority of women know they want change; however, most have not yet determined what kind of change will bring them the happiness and satisfaction that they know is missing from their lives, so they effect small partial change in a large number of areas of their lives.

It is instructive here to compare the National Survey's understanding of women's sexuality with that of Hite. By moving away from (apparently) simple behavioural acts, Hite's research shows that most of 'the action' in sexual and emotional terms does not focus on 'sex' in its specifically penetrational forms. Hite's approach, moreover, is one that permits women respondents to reply to questions in their own terms and words, making relevant and significant what *they* feel to be so and not what researchers assume this to be. There is, however, an issue concerning how these responses are textually represented and used, although overall it is almost impossible not to conclude that Hite's work provides a much richer picture of women's sexual and emotional lives and relationships than the narrow and genitally-focused one given in the National Survey, one which, moreover, demonstrates that for many women sexuality is less of a 'lifestyle' than it is a set of choices that can be made and re-made in different circumstances.

Some of the similarities between Hite's research and the substantive findings of 'Little Kinsey' are very noticeable: both perceive women's sexual dissatisfactions being both separate from their overall assessment of a relationship, but at the same time connected to it; both perceive many women's experiential dissent from 'sex' even while accepting the innateness and naturalness of this; both perceive men's focus on 'sex', their exclusion of emotional closeness, and their emotional dependence on women recast as women's dependence on them. However, *methodologically* even greater similarities are apparent, and it is these that I now discuss.

One of the most criticized aspects of Hite's research has concerned her sample, and, consequently, of whether and to what extent her results are generalizable and valid. Hite's sample is an achieved one; that is, it is the result of a very large number of people spontaneously and voluntarily writing responses and sending them to the project; it is not the product of a conventional approach, drawn by means of a sampling frame. Hite makes the point that the 'shape' or social characteristics of her resultant sample is not unrepresentative when compared with the characteristics of the total American population;[12] she also somewhat acidly and accurately notes that most conventional survey research actually uses unrepresentative samples, and that weighting a sample is the 'scientific' means of apparently making what is actually not representative appear as though it is by statistically manipulating an actually unrepresentative set of persons/data.[13] It may be doubted, however, whether anything less than a conventional random sample would have satisfied the critics, and very probably not even this if the findings she thereby produced were the same. That is, Hite's methodological departures from survey conventions provide a convenient stick with which to beat her, but the basic reason for the critical response is what are for many unpalatable and so unacceptable substantive results. It is interesting here to compare the criticisms of Hite's approach with those made of Mass-Observation. These seized upon similar aspects of the Mass-Observation approach to sampling, which was to make sure that a wide enough cross-section of people and situations were included for the researcher to gain an accurate insight into 'what was going on' with regard to the topic of investigation, not for precise targets of 'types of person' to be met or precise numerical results to be produced.[14] Mass-Observation's earlier *Britain and Her Birth-Rate* insisted that without the qualitative material the numerical results would be at best worthless, at worst highly misleading. The textual centrality in 'Little Kinsey' of extended quotations from respondents suggests that underpinning this also was a principled insistence on the central importance of people's own interpretations of their lives, with numerical analysis being a back-up rather than driving the analysis provided in the text.

Hite's study results, not from face-to-face interviewing using set questions with fixed choice answers, as is usual in surveys, but from an 'essay questionnaire' eliciting equally essay-like responses. It is interesting to compare this with the interviewing style adopted by Kinsey. Kinsey's interviews were extremely detailed, carried out over fairly lengthy periods of time spent with people, and were highly informal and completely non-judgmental and displayed an immense interest in people's lives and behaviours. From a considerably more conventional base, Kinsey's style of interviewing produced actually very similar responses to those of Hite, although, paradoxically perhaps, these were then analysed and placed within a set of academic textual conventions in which 'the numbers' dominated and the experiential richness was removed. 'Little Kinsey' is interestingly compared with both Hite and Kinsey. Here Mass-Observation used a conventional set question and fixed choice questionnaire, but the interviewers for the street sample part of the research then wrote detailed transcriptions of much of people's responses, with the questions constituting a trigger for these detailed responses rather than being merely a means of deriving numbers.

Hite presents her overall approach as '*a new methodological framework for analysis and presentation of data in mixed qualitative/quantitative research*',[15] and locates it within a critique of conventional science ideas about 'knowing', in particular the feminist variant of this critique.[16] The 'essay questionnaire' that Hite uses is one which asks for written responses to fairly long complex and interlinked questions, replies to which can be as long as the respondent feels appropriate. Quantification of these responses is seen by Hite as the simplest stage of an analytic approach that concentrates on first-person statements in order to explicate '*intricate categories of social patterns*'.[17] The actual process of analysis is described in all three Hite Reports.[18] It consists, first, of putting all the answers to each question on a chart, so that, by repeated reference to this, the 'categories' or patterns in the responses become apparent; and, second, of compiling a chart of the responses of each respondent so that an overall picture of them can be gained. Third, the text is then structured around the respondents's statements in the form of 'some', 'many', 'most' and representative quotations of each, with the 'some', 'many' and 'most' corresponding to particular percentage bands in the detailed numerical analysis provided in appendices. Such statements are then used to support a number of threads in the textual argument, which follow the categories or patterns of statements that Hite perceives in the responses from the respondents.

In basics, Hite's process of analysis is very similar to that adopted in the analysis of the 'Little Kinsey' data nearly 50 years earlier. Although there is no such comparable description of the analytic process that resulted in 'Little Kinsey', this can be recovered at least in outline from a comparison of the archived questionnaires, data analysis sheets and draft tables of frequencies and cross-tabulations against the final typescript. With 'Little Kinsey', a large number of tables of frequencies and of a variety of cross-tabulations were prepared by the researchers who worked on the questionnaires, and these were presented to the writer/analyst, who decided on their significance and relevance, sometimes noting comments regarding this on the sheets that contained the tables. The text of 'Little Kinsey' is written around thematic chapters and within each there is a main argumentative thread in which numbers of responses on particular topics are handled in the form of rhetorical glosses very similar to those used by Hite, 'some', 'most' and so forth.[19] This argumentative thread is in part structured through the very large number of quotations used, in part through the linking argument and commentary, again in a way similar to that used later by Hite.

It is extremely unlikely that Hite has any direct or even indirect knowledge of Mass-Observation's 1949 sex research. These coincidental similarities seem to have arisen because of parallel ideas about the need to retain the complexities of social life and behaviour within a survey approach. Once both 'a survey' and 'social complexity' are brought together, it is then highly likely that the nature of the questions asked, the means of recording answers to them, and the textual role of people's interpretations in their own words, will each come under scrutiny and the conventions either modified or more radically departed from. But as well as the similarities there are some interesting differences. 'Little Kinsey' is concerned with behaviour and attitude while Hite's research is concerned more with emotional response to behaviours, and Hite's research deals with very much larger numbers of people than does 'Little Kinsey' and asks more complex questions, for instance. However, the two differences that interest me most are, first, the differences produced by Hite centering women's point of view, which brings her work closer to *Britain and Her Birth-Rate* than to 'Little Kinsey'; and, second, the differences that result from the different textual and rhetorical strategies of Hite compared with the writer/analyst of 'Little Kinsey', which bring 'Little Kinsey' closer to the 'fragmented polyphony' of a postmodernist dis-authored text and Hite closer to the conventions of authorial authority.

Women As Revolutionary Agents of Change is the title of the 1993 compilation from the three Hite Reports;[20] its selections are harnessed to the theme of social change stemming from sexual change and women's part in producing this. Its culminating section is headed 'Women as revolutionary agents of change: to transform the culture with our values' and contains selections from Part V of *Women and Love*. Both this book's title and the arrangement of its contents make clear how, overall, the Hite Reports are to be read, that is, as a set of closely linked expositions on the central theme of women effecting change in their lives and in society more widely. Its 'Introduction' by Naomi Weisstein repeats this argument: '*We seem to be living in a time of radical shift . . . Women all over the United States have come to some very important conclusions; indeed, their whole perspective on the world seems to be changing . . . women defining themselves emotionally . . . on their own terms, saying goodbye to an allegiance to 'male' cultural values . . . This debate is in part about what 'women's revolution' will mean to the society: if we change our status, will the whole society be changed, thereby transformed?'*[21] While Weisstein leaves this question of social transformation open, as indicated by the interrogatory question mark here, Hite's own text is much less cautious. Its final sub-sections are in Hite's own words, quotations from respondents are almost entirely absent, and the message is quite clear: women's resistance is the beginning of change that will result in an alternative social system and a new social contract, *'not only with each other but also with the planet and the other creatures who share the earth'.*[22] This process of change is one that Hite sees as the continuation and development of two previous phases of change occurring since at least the mid-nineteenth century, of equal rights, followed by joining 'male' activities, with her research detailing the third phase, of women consolidating their different values; the fourth phase, which Hite perceives as already underway, is to 'change the culture' by means of women's values, to transform it.

Hite centres women's point of view about sex throughout the three substantive Reports on her research, including when her respondents are men by focusing on men's emotional and relational ties with women. Her analysis has followed key topics and themes merely, apparently, as these have been presented by successive groups of respondents to the Hite questionnaires over what is a considerable period of time in social research terms, from 1972 until 1986. Hite sees her analysis as less her promoting a particular – and political – point of view, and more her 'giving voice' to women's own point of view. Accusations of its 'bias', she insists, stem from both the newness of this 'voice' being heard and the rejection of what it says because it departs from the dominant male-centred 'knowledge' about such issues.[23] This is similar to the approach of *Britain and Her Birth-Rate*, and with similar criticisms being made of it: seeing the world from the viewpoint of women produces knowledge that is radically different from how 'reality' has been previously seen – that is, only from the viewpoint of men – while seeing from women's viewpoint on social life is construed as biased (presumptively, doing so from men's is not). The difference is that Hite sees sex as causative of these other changes, while *Britain and Her Birth-Rate* does not.

Hite's research certainly constitutes an interesting departure from modern survey convention in a number of ways, not least regarding her concern with meaning, feeling and emotion. As all three Hite Reports note, this area of social life is the hardest thing to get at in a survey approach. Insofar as centring 'the numbers' necessitates removing the nuances of meaning and feeling, then the de-centring of 'numbers' in Hite's research, as in 'Little Kinsey', enables people's emotional responses to sexual and related behaviours to be 'heard' within these research reports. There is an interesting difference here between Hite and 'Little Kinsey', however, one that stems from what I earlier termed the 'failure' of 'Little Kinsey' to hear what dissatisfied women were saying. In Hite's work, the texts of the three Reports are replete with 'voices', the statements and ideas and arguments of the respondents, women respondents, and men respondents 'speaking' to themes deemed important by the women. But there is in my view a clear and dominant authorial 'voice' within them all, the voice or inscription of Shere Hite, while the rhetorical strategy of 'Little Kinsey', as I have argued, leads to both the presence and the dispersal of such authorial authority. Hite argues that her texts are marked by the complete separation of data and statement from interpretation, that her textual 'voice' appears only in relation to interpretation.[24] In my view this is really not convincing, for it begs the crucial question of 'who selects', who selects in what is deemed significant and interesting, around what topics and themes, and using what quoted passages from respondents' writings. That is, there is both an acknowledged authorial presence – 'I interpret, but you have the data' – and a denied researcher presence – 'I select the data'.

Hite's critique of 'science', I conclude, is a partial one that stops short of acknowledging central arguments in feminist social science writing concerned with reflexivity and epistemology. It is highly unlikely that Hite is unaware of this very powerful and influential strand in feminist work; the partiality of her critique results, presumably, because Hite, like other feminist proponents of a modified version of the survey approach, wishes to claim generalizability, validity, acceptability, truth and science for her research, a survey made 'better science' by its feminism.[25] That is, Hite makes major knowledge-claims from her work, about the entire course of social change in American society, and she sees it as constituting a better and superior form of producing certain knowledge about social life than is provided by the masculinist form of 'big science'. In the light of the vociferous, and often unfair, criticisms of Hite's work, books, appearance and public presentations of self, it is tempting to treat her as a kind of martyr to an anti-feminist backlash. My own view is that these mainstream criticisms are a predictable response to her attempt to 'join the boys' while also trying to take some of their methodological toys from them, and that an overall assessment should look at not only the substantive 'findings' of Hite's research but also its methodological innovations and epistemological problematics.

The substantive results of Hite's research constitute an interesting confirmation of the broad general picture provided in much earlier work, including 'Little Kinsey'. The methodological innovations are in my view much less innovative than Hite and her supporters propose. Many other researchers, before, during and after Hite's researches, have mixed quantitative and qualitative forms of investigation and data; and 'Little Kinsey' did so over 30 years earlier in Hite's own area of sexual behaviour and sexual attitude. The main methodological innovation in Hite's work is its removal of 'the numbers' from rhetorical and textual centrality, resulting in 'a survey' that is different in form and function from the dominant post-war version of what this should be. Consequently, it is hardly surprising that relegating 'the numbers' in this way should occasion criticism and rejection from those who are 'believers' in the current survey movement in the social sciences. Hite's choice has been to counter these criticisms by invoking 'better science', taking on and countering conventional views about representative sampling and the relationship between numerical and interpretational forms of analysis of survey data. Interestingly, however, she has not chosen to challenge the notion of 'science' in any fundamental way, remaining firmly within a science epistemological frame with regard to the generalizability and validity of her work and the knowledge-claims that can be made from it.

It is in relation to epistemological debates and ideas that Hite's work appears shakiest. It is useful here to consider what removing 'the numbers' from textual centrality does in terms of the knowledge-claims of 'science'. It removes claims to certain and precise knowledge – that is, the very essence of 'science' in conventional formulations – to the textual sidelines, and places at the centre a rhetorical strategy that revolves around levels of interpretation: the interpretations of the respondents, and the interpretations of the researcher/author. Thus, Hite's approach both seeks to make exactly the kind of certain, and predictive, knowledge-claims about the social world that the precise, definite, numbers of science are seen to permit, *and* at the same time it relegates the prime means of doing so to an entirely subordinate evidential position. However interesting, however illuminating, however insightful, interpretation is by definition neither definite nor precise. By its very nature interpretation is concerned with difference, nuance, complexity, and the existence of competing interpretational claims: all the features of social life which mean that making knowledge-claims is a highly uncertain business. It is the role of numbers in stripping away difference and complexity that constitutes their seduction and their apparent empowering of those who employ them. But once interpretation is allowed in the door to take centre place on the page, then researchers and writers move into a different epistemological frame. Hite notes and applauds a feminist hermeneutics,[26] but at the same time she attempts to retain all the status and acceptability of scientific foundationalism for her work.

One of the most interesting analytic features of Hite's research is its attempt to research notions of change, looking at personal change and its links with wider social change, and exploring sexual change and how it might underpin aspects of the broader gamut of economic and political change in social life. It is this analytic theme of change and its connections with methodological issues and strategies in relation to the sex survey more widely that I now turn to, as the concluding feature of my broad overview of the sex survey tradition.

Notes

1   For a brief selection, see here: Cartledge and Ryan (1983); Holly (1989); Jackson (1982); Segal (1994); Sherfey (1972); Stimpson and Person (1980); Vance (1989), Wilkinson and Kitzinger (1993), Wittig (1992).

2   These ideas have been widely debated in academic feminism, and my own work is a part of this discourse. For useful discussions of the epistemological aspects of a feminist engagement with 'science', presenting a variety of different but equally feminist viewpoints, see Bordo (1986, 1987); Harding (1986, 1991); Rose (1993); Schiebinger (1994); and Stanley and Wise (1993).

3   I began my research career in the later 1960s as a junior researcher working on large-scale datasets in the context of new towns research; more recently in the later 1980s I was Director of the Manchester-based part of the ESRC's 'Social Change and Economic Life' Initiative research in Rochdale and responsible for its two surveys, one a Kish grid derived random sample, the other a 'household' sub-sample of this, as well as of other related studies.

4   See here Stanley and Wise (1979) and (1993) for an 'early' and a 'late' exposition of this view.

5   This is the viewpoint argued in the introduction to Stanley (1990b), a collection of theoretically and methodologically divergent feminist researches, but all of which share a concern with epistemological issues and problematics.

6   See here the overview of feminist survey work and accompanying references in Reinharz (1992), pp. 76–94.

7   Hite (1974) *Sexual Honesty* p. 2.

8   Hite (1987) *Women and Love* p. 4.

9   Hite (1987) p. 147.

10   Hite (1987) pp. 649–772.

11   Hite (1987) p. 650, p. 653.

12   Hite (1987) pp. 1058–9; see also (1976) pp. 23–55; (1987) pp. 1055–78.

13   Hite (1987) pp. 777–8.

14   The most succinct and convincing exposition of this Mass-Observation approach is to be found in *Britain and Her Birth-Rate* (Mass-Observation 1945, pp. 7–15, and 208–44). It defines what is 'a good sample' around achieving knowledge of trends in people's ideas and behaviours, and not the absolute figures aimed at by the conventional sample survey. This report insists, *'The whole report is essentially interpretive, and without the mass of qualitative material available the numerical results would be at best so superficial as to be of little value, at worst would seem to lead to conclusions which the verbatim material shows to be false'* (p. 208).

15   Hite (1987) p. 773.

16   Hite (1987) pp. 769–77.

17   Hite (1987) p. 774.

18   See here Hite (1976) *Female Sexuality* pp. 51–2; (1981) *Male Sexuality* pp. 1057–60; and (1987) *Women and Love* pp. 779–782.

19   However, my comparison of these textual statements against the many archived tables from this project suggests that the use of such terms in 'Little Kinsey' is very much less precise than Hite's.

20   Hite (1993) *Women As Revolutionary Agents of Change.*

21   Weisstein (1993) p. 12.

22   Hite (1993) p. 410.

23   Hite (1987) pp. 1059–60.

24   Hite (1987) p. 780.

25   See here Kelly (1988) for another influential example of a feminist survey that seeks to make the same kind of 'better science' knowledge-claims.

26   See here Hite (1987) pp. 770–3.

Chapter 9

Sex Changes? Sex Surveys and Social Change

The existence and development of changes in the way that people think about and decide to live their emotional and sexual relationships is of profound importance to us all. If such change is indeed occurring – and I return to this point – then this would affect social life in all manner of ways. It would affect how people think of their sexuality (including of themselves thinking sexually about others), how they think about 'sex' and what this is seen to consist of and with whom under what kind of conditions, what role is given to personal sexual pleasure within emotionally committed relationships, how emotional commitment itself is evaluated, how and if marriage remains a part of people's lives, what the status and roles of partners will be, whether children are seen as a feature of partnerships and who is seen to be responsible for their care. And, because of these things, it would also affect women's and men's participation in the labour market, domestic divisions of labour, the role of employment in people's lives, caring for the sick or disabled or elderly, the demand for child care and the role of public provision, public policy concerned with employment legislation, divorce, custody, and a wide range of other matters. This list could go on almost infinitely; however, the main point has been made, which is that 'sexual change' could not occur in a vacuum, for the sexual is a part of the social not least because it is complexly linked to other aspects of social life in a wide variety of ways.

Given this interrelationship of the sexual and the social, defining what constitutes 'sexual change' and exploring why it might occur, deciding how to measure it, and discerning when it is happening, are, individually and collectively, not simple matters. This is not least because, as I discussed earlier, merely defining 'sex' is itself both complex and highly contentious; and these contentious complexities are of course multiplied when 'change' is brought into the picture. Moreover, 'change' is not unitary: for example, is the change personal, sectional (i.e. affecting particular classes, or genders, or regions, and so forth) or more general? Is it short-run or long run? Does the change occur progressively in some areas of life but is then compensated for regressively in other areas? Does it occur continuously, or are there discontinuities, with periods of change being followed by periods (of shorter, equal, or longer, length) of stasis? And so on.

The National Survey is based on the conviction that what is required is an accurate set of information about 'sexual attitudes and sexual lifestyles' – that is, about what is happening sexually at the moment – so that this can then act as the baseline for discerning and measuring future change in the area of sex and sexuality. On one level this is a strategically sensible way of approaching the complexities of researching sexual change. However, as I have already discussed, the National Survey rigorously removes everything concerned with meaning and feeling from its research and it is thereby prevented from understanding sexual behaviour itself, for the 'same' sexual act can mean different things and so can be experienced very differently. And, relatedly, as Mass-Observation's *Britain and Her Birth-Rate* and 'Little Kinsey', as well as Shere Hite's research, have each shown, 'change' may be not very discernible when looking at and measuring sexual *behaviour*, but may be shown to be obviously important when focusing on sexual *meanings, emotions and feelings*.

Surveys are good ways of carrying out relatively simple research tasks, counting behaviour being prime here. However, the National Survey in my view has defined the range of sexual behaviour with which it is concerned too narrowly and in ways that are gender-problematic. Hite avoids this problem by not proposing researcher-provided definitions at all; she also centres the issue of behavioural complexity by recognizing that a range of meanings and feelings for the 'same' behaviour can exist, and also by emphasizing that such variant meanings may become an important issue in sexual and emotional relationships. However, these strategic decisions, along with her analytic concerns, then bring Hite up against the complexities of defining and measuring sexual change and discerning its relationship to other aspects of social change. Seemingly, Hite's response to such issues is to assume that the existence of widespread personal dissatisfaction means both that the desire for change will result in actual 'on the ground' sexual and relational changes, and also that these changes will then necessarily result in wider social and economic change. However, the existence of widespread dissatisfaction and short-run personal change need not necessarily result in either longer-term personal change nor short- nor long-term wider social and economic change. Hite seems to think that widespread short-term personal sexual change *necessarily* acts as some kind of causal agent. This *may* have a causal affect on other aspects of social and sexual life; however, its causal status has to be demonstrated, not merely assumed.

Assumptions about sexual and social change are to be found in most of the sex surveys discussed earlier as well as in Hite's work. In a way, the passing of time is almost seen to be in itself a necessary producer of sexual and social change; thus an entire generation of teenagers is assumed to be more promiscuous that the previous one, attitudes to a wide range of sexual behaviour are assumed to be more liberal and progressive, and so on. The factor that permits such research assumptions is more often than not that members of research samples say that such change has occurred. However, this is to rely upon people's opinions and, as 'Little Kinsey' forcibly reminds us, opinion is often very much removed from people's first-hand experience and knowledge and is all the more unreliable for being so.

Perception of 'change' can be an artefact of the process of research, and I think this is true of Hite's research. By its centring of 'women's point of view', something different about social and sexual life is shown, something which departs from conventional – and male – knowledge. It is perhaps paradoxical that it has been primarily feminist research which has 'normalized' male sexuality by displacing it from the centre of knowledge and replacing it with the relational focus that 'women's point of view' is concerned with. Looked at like this, it is by no means surprising that the Hite Reports 'reveal' dissatisfaction and change; it is interesting to contemplate the possibility that research carried out at any point in time – say the 1830s, or the 1880s, or the 1910s, or the 1940s, or the 1990s – which centres women's lives, experiences and understandings might show this. That is, perhaps in western societies a comparison of women's sexual and emotional lives, at least for the last 150 years or so, might reveal a widespread pattern of short-run personal and sexual change: life as a learning experience in which women effect change in order to exert some measure of control. I should perhaps emphasize that this is not an argument I am myself making. I introduce it to make the point that the social and sexual behaviour that Mass-Observation's and Hite's researches have focused on can be explained in ways other than that assumed by Hite, indeed assumed by Mass-Observation also, concerning widespread long-term social and economic change for the whole society.

The survey research I have discussed is in fact concerned with stasis and change in *western* societies and largely for *white* Britons and Americans; in addition, and in spite of the National Survey's inclusion of homosexual behaviour and partners as a 'lifestyle' and Hite's recognition of a spectrum of sexual feelings and involvements, these researches are also predominately *heterosexually* oriented and concerned. It seems to me axiomatic that any satisfactory attempt to come to grips with sexual and social change must take into account the specificity of western societies; the fact that western populations are not exclusively and in some local cases not predominantly white; and that sexual behaviour is for many people increasingly experienced as a choice, one that is not necessarily or exclusively or permanently heterosexual, and once emotions are brought into the picture then sexuality and its choices become even more complex.

It remains to be seen whether the sex survey can be developed in ways that make it more satisfactorily responsive to the issues raised here about sexual change and whether linked wider social and economic change is occurring. It may be, as 'Little Kinsey' and Hite both imply, that 'less and better' science is needed in order to do so. 'The survey' and its canonical status as 'science' is, as I have argued, largely a post-war development. 'Little Kinsey' ambivalently both challenged and reinforced these claims at their moment of origin, Hite's work does so later when this status has become largely taken-for-granted as 'true fact'. Their attempts to modify scientific convention do so to the point where the result is hardly 'a survey' at all; it remains to be seen whether either will feature significantly in future accounts of the sex survey tradition. But whatever, the canonical claims of the sex survey will surely be looked at with a more critical eye as a consequence of their work.

References

ABRAMS, Mark (1951) *Social Surveys and Social Action*, London, Heinemann.

ALLEN, Clifford (1940) *The Sexual Perversions and Anomalies*, Oxford, Oxford University Press.

ALLEN, Clifford (1950) *The Grammar of Marriage*, London, Heinemann.

ALLEN, Clifford (1952) *Modern Discoveries in Medical Psychology*, London, Macmillan.

ALLEN, Clifford (1958) *Homosexuality: Its Nature, Causation and Treatment*, London, Staples Press.

ALLEN, Clifford (1962) *A Textbook of Psychosexual Disorders*,Oxford,, Oxford University Press.

BARTLETT, Frederick, GINSBERG, Morris, LINDGREN, Ethel and THOU-LESS, Ralph (Eds) (1939) *The Study of Society*, London, Routledge & Kegan Paul.

BIBBY, Cyril (1944) *Sex Education: A Guide for Parents, Teachers and Youth Leaders*, London, Macmillan.

BIBBY, Cyril (1946a) *Health Education*, London, Heinemann.

BIBBY Cyril (1946b) *How Life is Handed On*, London, Heinemann.

BLOOME, David, SHERIDAN, Dorothy and STREET, Brian (1994) 'Reading Mass-Observation writing', *Auto/Biography*, **2**(2), pp.7–38

BORDO, Susan (1986) 'The Cartesian masculinisation of thought', *Signs*, **11**, pp. 439–55.

BORDO, Susan (1987) *The Flight to Objectivity: Essays on Cartesianism and Culture*, New York, SUNY Press.

BRIGHTON OURSTORY PROJECT (1992) *Daring Hearts: Lesbian and Gay Lives of 50s and 60s Brighton*, Brighton, Queenspark Books.

BULMER, Martin (1982a) 'The development of sociology and of empirical social research in Britain' in BULMER, M. (Ed.) *Essays on the History of British Sociological Research*, Cambridge, Cambridge University Press, pp.3–36.

BULMER, Martin (Ed.) (1982b) *Essays on the History of British Sociological Research*, Cambridge, Cambridge University Press.

BULMER, Martin, BALES, Kevin and SKLAR, Kathryn (Eds) (1991) *The Social*

Survey in Historical Perspective 1880–1940, Cambridge, Cambridge University Press.

BUNN, Margaret (1943) 'Mass-Observation: a comment on *People in Production'*, *Manchester School*, **31**, pp. 24–37.

CARTLEDGE, Sue and RYAN, Joanna (Eds) (1983) *Sex and Love: New Thoughts on Old Contradictions*, London, The Women's Press.

CHAPMAN, Dennis (1955) *The Home and Social Status*, London, Routledge.

CHESSER, Eustace (1941) *Love Without Fear*, London, Rich & Cowan.

CHESSER, Eustace (1946a, 1957 revised version) *Marriage and Freedom*, London, Pan Books.

CHESSER, Eustace with DAWE Zoe (1946b) *The Practice of Sex Education: A Plain Guide for Parents and Teachers*, London, Medical Publications.

CHESSER, Eustace (1949a) *Grow Up – and Live*, Harmondsworth, Penguin.

CHESSER, Eustace (1949b) *Sexual Behaviour, Normal and Abnormal*, London, Medical Publications.

CHESSER, Eustace with DAVEY, Charles and GORER Geoffrey (1961) *Teenage Morals*, London, Councils and Education Press.

CHESSER, Eustace (1965) *The Sexual, Marital and Family Relationships of the English Woman*, London, Hutchinson.

CROSS, Gary (Ed.) (1990)*Worktowners at Blackpool: Mass-Observation and popular leisure in the 1930s*, London, Routledge.

DAVENPORT-HINES, Richard (1990) *Sex, Death and Punishment*, London, Collins.

ENGLAND, Len (1949) 'Little Kinsey: an outline of sex attitudes in Britain', *Public Opinion Quarterly*, **13**, pp.587–600.

ENGLAND, Len (1950) 'A British sex survey' *International Journal of Sexology*, **3**, pp.148–54.

FIELD, Julia and WADSWORTH, Jane (1989) 'Developing the methodology for a national survey of sexual attitudes and lifestyles' in *Joint Centre for Survey Methods Newsletter*: 'Issues in researching sexual behaviour', **10**, 1, pp.5–8.

FIRTH, Raymond (1939) 'An anthropologist's view of Mass-Observation', *Sociological Review*, **31**, pp.166–93.

GAGNON, John and SIMON, William (1973) *Sexual Conduct*, Chicago, Aldine.

GORER, Geoffrey (1955) *Exploring English Character*, London, Cresset Press.

GORER, Geoffrey (1971) *Sex and Marriage in England Today*, London, Nelson.

HALL, Lesley (1991) *Hidden Anxieties: Male Sexuality, 1900–1950*, Oxford, Polity Press.

HALL CARPENTER ARCHIVES (1989a) *Inventing Ourselves: Lesbian Life Stories*, London, Routledge.

HALL CARPENTER ARCHIVES (1989b) *Walking After Midnight: Gay Men's Life Stories*, London, Routledge.

HARDING, Sandra (1986) *The Science Question in Feminism*, Milton Keynes, Open University Press.

HARDING, Sandra (Ed.) (1987) *Feminism and Methodology*, Buckingham, Open University Press.

HARDING, Sandra (1991) *Whose Science, Whose Knowledge?*, Milton Keynes, Open University Press.

HARRISSON, Tom (1937) *Savage Civilisation*, London, Gollancz.

HARRISSON, Tom (1947) 'The future of sociology *Pilot Papers*, spring 1947.

HARRISSON, Tom and MADGE Charles (1939) *Britain, by Mass-Observation*, Harmondsworth, Penguin; reprinted by The Cressett Library, London.

HASTE, Cate (1992) *Rules of Desire*, London, Chatto and Windus.

HITE, Shere (1974) *Sexual Honesty*, New York, Warner.

HITE, Shere (1976) *The Hite Report on Female Sexuality*, London, Pandora Press.

HITE, Shere (1981) *The Hite Report on Male Sexuality,* London, Optima.

HITE, Shere (1987) *The Hite Report on Women and Love*, Penguin, Harmondsworth.

HITE, Shere (1993) *Women as Revolutionary Agents of Change*, London, Sceptre/Hodder and Stoughton.

HOLLY, Lesley (Ed.) (1989) *Girls and Sexuality*, Milton Keynes, Open University Press.

HUBBACK, Eva (1945) *Population Facts and Policies*, London, Allen and Unwin.

HUBBACK, Eva (1947) *The Population of Britain*, Harmondsworth, Penguin.

HUMPHRIES, Steve (1988) *A Secret World of Sex*, London, Sidgwick & Jackson.

JACKSON, Margaret (1994) *The Real Facts of Life*, London, Taylor & Francis.

JACKSON, Stevi (1982) *Childhood and Sexuality*, Oxford, Blackwell.

JAHODA, Marie (1938) 'Review of Mass-Observation and of *May 12*', *Sociological Review*, **30**, pp.208–9.

JAHODA-LAZERSFELD, Marie and ZEISEL, Hans (1933, 1972 translation) *Marienthal*, London, Tavistock Publications.

JEFFREYS, Sheila (1985) *The Spinster and Her Enemies: Feminism and Sexuality 1880–1930* London, Pandora Press.

JEFFREYS, Sheila (1990) *Anticlimax: A feminist perspective on the sexual revolution*, London, The Women's Press.

JENNINGS, Humphrey and MADGE, Charles (1937) *May 12: Mass-Observation Day-Surveys*, London, Faber & Faber.

JOHNSON, Anne, WADSWORTH, Jane, WELLINGS, Kaye, BRADSHAW, Sally and FIELD Julia (1992) 'Sexual lifestyles and HIV risk', *Nature*, **360**, pp.410–12.

JOHNSON, Anne, WADSWORTH, Jane, WELLINGS, Kaye and FIELD, Julia (1994) *Sexual Attitudes and Lifestyles*, Oxford, Blackwell Scientific.

JOINT CENTRE FOR SURVEY METHODS NEWSLETTER (1989) 'Issues in researching sexual behaviour', **10**, 1.

KELLY, Liz (1988) *Surviving Sexual Violence*, Cambridge, Polity Press.

KEOGH, Peter (1994) 'Swelling the numbers', *The Pink Paper* 4 February, p.13

KINSEY, Alfred (1948) *Sexual Behaviour in the Human Male*, New York, W.B. Saunders.

KINSEY, Alfred (1953) *Sexual Behaviour in the Human Female*, New York, W.B. Saunders.

LENNON, Kathleen and WHITFORD, Margeret (Eds) (1994) *Knowing the Difference: Feminist Perspectives in Epistemology*, London, Routledge.

LOWE, Adolf (1935) *Economics and Society*, London, Allen & Unwin.

MACE, David (1944) *The Facts About Venereal Disease*, London, Alliance of Honour.

MACE, David (1946) *Does Sexual Morality Matter?*, London, Rich & Cowan.

MACE, David (1971) *The Christian Response to the Sexual Revolution*, London, Lutterworth Press.

MADGE, Charles (1943) *Wartime Pattern of Savings and Spending National Institute of Economic and Social Research Occasional Paper IV*, Cambridge, Cambridge University Press.

MADGE, Charles and HARRISSON, Tom (1937) *Mass-Observation*, London, Muller.

MADGE, Charles and HARRISSON, Tom (1938) *First Year's Work*, London, Lindsay Drummond.

MALINOWSKI, Bronislaw (1938) 'A nation-wide intelligence service' in MADGE, Charles and HARRISSON, Tom (Eds) *First Year's Work*, London, Lindsay Drummond, pp.81–121.

MARSH, Catherine (1982a) *The Survey Method*, London, Allen & Unwin.

MARSH, Catherine (1982b) 'Informants, respondents and citizens' in BULMER, Martin (Ed.) *Essays on the History of British Sociological Research*, Cambridge, Cambridge University Press, pp.206–227.

MARSHALL, Thomas (1937) 'Is Mass-Observation moonshine?', *The Highway*, **30**, pp. 48–50.

MASS-OBSERVATION (1943a) *War Factory*, London, Hutchinson; written by Celia Fremlin and reprinted by The Cressett Library, London.

MASS-OBSERVATION (1943b) *The Pub and the People*, London, Gollancz; reprinted by The Cressett Library, London.

MASS-OBSERVATION (1945) *Britain and Her Birth-Rate*, London, Advertising Standards Guild.

MITCHISON, Naomi (1985) *Among You Taking Notes: The Wartime Diary of Naomi Mitchison 1935–1945, London, Gollancz.*

MORGAN, David and STANLEY, Liz (Eds) (1993) *Debates in Sociology*, Manchester, Manchester University Press.

MORT Frank (1987) *Dangerous Sexualities: Medico-Moral Politics in England Since 1830*, London, Routledge.

NEILD, Suzanne and PEARSON, Rosalind (1992) *Women Like Us*, London, The Women's Press.

OESER, Oscar (1937) 'Methods and assumptions of fieldwork', *British Journal of Psychology*, **27**, pp.343–63.

OESER, Oscar (1939) 'The value of team work and functional penetration as methods in social investigation' in BARTLETT, Frederick *et al.* (Eds) *Study of Society*, London, Routledge & Kegan Paul, pp.402–17.

PEAR, T.H. (1939) 'Some problems and topics of contemporary social psychology' in BARTLETT, Frederick *et al.* (Eds) *The Study of Society*, London, Routledge & Kegan Paul, pp.1–23.

PENELOPE, Julia and WOLFE, Susan (1980 and 1989) *The Original Coming Out Stories*, Freedom, California, The Crossing Press.

PILGRIM TRUST (1938) *Men Without Work*, Cambridge, Cambridge University Press.

REINHARZ, Shulamit (1992) *Feminist Methods in Social Research*, New York, Oxford University Press.

ROSE, Hilary (1993) *Love, Power and Knowledge: Towards a feminist transformation of the sciences*, Cambridge, Polity Press.

SCHIEBINGER, Londa (1994) *Nature's Body: sexual politics and the making of modern science*, London, Pandora Press.

SCHOFIELD, Michael (1965) *The Sexual Behaviour of Young People*, Harmondsworth, Penguin.

SCHOFIELD, Michael (1968) *The Sexual Behaviour of Young Adults*, London, Allen Lane.

SCHOFIELD, Michael (1976) *Promiscuity*, London, Gollancz.

SEGAL, Lynne (1994) *Straight Sex*, London, Virago Press.

SHERFEY, Mary Jane (1972) *The Nature and Evolution of Female Sexuality*, New York, Random House.

SHERIDAN, Dorothy (1992) 'Ordinary hard-working folk: volunteer writers in Mass-Observation, 1937–50 and 1981–91', *Feminist Praxis*, **37/38**, pp.1–34.

SHERIDAN Dorothy (1993) 'Writing to the Archive: Mass-Observation as autobiography', *Sociology*, **27**, pp.27–40.

SLATER, Eliot and WOODSIDE, Moya (1951) *Patterns of Marriage: A Study of Marital Relationships in the Urban Working Class*, London, Cassell.

STANLEY, Liz (1990a) 'The archaeology of a 1930s Mass-Observation project', *University of Manchester Occasional Papers in Sociology*, no.27.

STANLEY, Liz (Ed.) (1990b) *Feminist Praxis: Theory, Method and Epistemology in Feminist Sociology*, London, Routledge.

STANLEY, Liz (1992) 'The economics of everyday life: a Mass-Observation project in Bolton', *North West Labour History Journal*, **17**, pp.95–102.

STANLEY, Liz (1995) "Little Kinsey' and its methods of investigation and analysis' unpublished paper.

STANLEY, Liz and WISE, Sue (1979) 'Feminist research, feminist consciousness and experiences of sexism', *Women's Studies International Forum*, **2**, pp.359–74.

STANLEY Liz and WISE Sue (1990) 'Method, methodology and epistemology in feminist research processes' in STANLEY, Liz (Ed.) *Feminist Praxis: Theory, Method and Epistemology in Feminist Sociology*, London, Routledge, pp.20–64.

STANLEY, Liz and WISE, Sue (1993) *Breaking Out Again: Feminist Ontology and Epistemology*, London, Routledge.

STIMPSON, Catharine and PERSON, Ethel (Eds) (1980) *Women, Sex and Sexuality*, Chicago, Chicago University Press.

SUMMERFIELD, Penny (1992) 'Mass-Observation on women at work in the Second World War' *Feminist Praxis*, **37/38**, pp.35–49.

TATCHELL, Peter (1993) 'Where are the missing millions?', *Gay Times*, January, **172**, pp.14–15.

References

VANCE, Carole (Ed.) (1989) *Pleasure and Danger: Exploring Female Sexuality*, London, Pandora Press.

VERNON, P.E. (1939) 'Questionnaires, attitude tests, and rating scales' in BARTLETT, Frederick GINSBERG, M, LINGREN E, and THOULESS R, (Eds) *The Study of Society*, London, Routledge & Kegan Paul, pp.199–229.

WADSWORTH, Jane and JOHNSON, Anne (1991) 'Measuring sexual behaviour', *Journal Royal Statistical Society*, **154**, pp.367–70.

WEEKS, Jeffrey (1981/1989) *Sex, Politics and Society*, London, Longman.

WEINBERG, Martin (Ed.) (1976) *Sex Research: Studies from the Kinsey Institute*, New York, Oxford University Press.

WEISSTEIN, Naomi (1993) 'An introduction to the Hite Reports: theory and importance' in HITE Shere *Women as Revolutionary Agents of Change*, London, Sceptre/Hodden & Stoughton, pp.1–13.

WELLINGS, Kaye, FIELD, Julia, WADSWORTH, Jane, JOHNSON, Anne and BRADSHAW, Sallie (1990) 'Sexual lifestyles under scrutiny', *Nature*, **348**, November, pp.276–8.

WELLINGS, Kaye, FIELD, Julia, JOHNSON, Anne and WADSWORTH, Jane (1994) *Sexual Behaviour in Britain*, Harmondsworth, Penguin.

WELLS, Alan (1936) 'Social surveys and sociology', *Sociological Review*, **28**, pp.274–94.

WILKINSON, Sue and KITZINGER, Celia (Eds) (1993) *Heterosexuality, A Reader*, London, Sage.

WITTIG, Monique (1992) *The Straight Mind and Other Essays*, New York, Harvester.

YOUNG, Terence (1934) *Becontree and Dagenham: A Report*, London, Pilgrim Trust Becontree Social Survey Committee.

Subject Index

Abdication crisis 11
adultery 25, 48-9, 58, 132-42

Beacontree 24
'believers' 221, 230
Blackpool, *see* Mass-Observation
Bolton, *see* Mass-Observation
British Institute of Public Opinion (BIPO)
  24, 30, 208-9, 210
British Market Research Bureau Ltd, *see*
  Mass-Observation Ltd

change 6, 35, 39, 43-4, 62, 63, 219, 225,
  228-9, 231, 233-6; *see also* Hite
  Reports
  role of causality in 6, 42-4, 234-5
Churchtown, *see* Mass-Observation
contraception 25, 39, 95-110, 215, 216

Dagenham 24
divorce, *see* 'Little Kinsey', separation and
  divorce

'Economics of Everyday Life' project, *see*
  Mass-Observation
ethnography 5, 208

facts of life, the 25, 74-85, 215
feminism 4, 6-7, 10, 42, 221, 222
  feminist epistemologies 21, 209, 222,
  230-1
  feminist methodology 9, 230
  feminist sex surveys 221-32
  methodological canon within 222

Gallop, *see* British Institute of Public
  Opinion

heterosexuality 29, 41, 45, 47, 60, 61-2,
  215, 218, 235
Hite Reports 53, 221-32, 234-5; *see also*
  Hite, Shere
  conceptualisation of 'sex' 224
  epistemological shakiness 230-1
  findings 223-5, 230
  and male sexuality 224-5
  methodological approach 227-8
  questionnaire 223
  sample 226
  and science 230
  and sexual-social change 228-9, 231,
  234, 235
  and women's point of view 223-4, 225,
  229
HIV/AIDS 49-50
homosexuality 25, 45, 46-7, 50-2, 60, 194,
  199-203, 211, 235; *see also* 'Little
  Kinsey, lesbianism

Left Book Club 11
lesbianism 45, 52-3, 60, 224, 235; *see also*
  homosexuality
'Little Kinsey' 3-10, 21-4, 25, 65-203, 209,
  211-20, 226-8, 229, 230
  advisors to 5, 22, 71-2, 73
  analytic process 227-8
  birth control 95-110; *see also* contraception
  divorce 123-31; *see also* separation
  and divorce
  extra-marital sex 132-42; *see also*
  adultery, sex before marriage
  in history of sex research 37-8
  homosexual groups 25, 199-203, 211;
  see also homosexuality

Author Index

Abrams, Mark 30, 35, 209, 210
Adams Mary 14
Allen, Clifford 5, 10
Aristotle 77

Baldamus Wilheim 19
Bales, Kevin, *see* Bulmer, Martin, Skales,
    Kevin, and Sklar, Kathryn
Bartlett, Frederick 17, 207, 209
Bibby, Cyril 5, 10, 73
Block, Ivan 154
Bloome, David, Sheridan, Dorothy, and
    Street, Brian 18
Bordo, Susan 232
Bowen-Partington W. 77
Brighton Ourstory Project 56
Bulmer, Martin 18, 209; *see also* Bulmer,
    Martin, Skales, Kevin, and Sklar,
    Kathryn
Bulmer, Martin, Skales, Kevin, and Sklar,
    Kathryn 209
Bunn, Margaret 14, 17

Carpenter, Edward 85
Cartledge, Sue and Ryan, Joanna 231
Chapman, Dennis 16
Chesser, Eustace 36-7, 40-4, 45, 46, 49,
    54, 59-62; *see also* Chesser,
    Eustace, and Dawe, Zoe, *The Sexual,*
    Marital and Family Relationships of
    the English Woman
Chesser, Eustace, and Dawe, Zoe 54
Cross, Gary 10, 27

Daily Mirror 11, 122
Darwin, Charles 13

Davenport-Hines, Richard 53

Ellis, Havelock 76
England, Len 15, 21, 22, 23, 24, 26, 27,
    203, 211, 219; *see also* 'Little
    Kinsey'

Ferraby, John 15, 27
Field, Julia, and Wadsworth, Jane 55; *see*
    also National Survey of Sexual
    Attitudes and Lifestyles
Firth, Raymond 14, 17
Florence, Philip Sargant 19, 208
Fowler L. N. 77
Fremlin, Celia 18
Freud, Sigmund 77

Gagnon, John, and Simon, William 64
Ginsberg, Morris 17
Gollancz, Victor 17
Gorer, Geoffrey 37, 47-9, 55, 59-62; *see*
    also Sex and Marriage in England
    Today
Gray, Dr 77

Haire, Norman 76
Hall Carpenter Archives 56
Hall, Leslie 37, 53, 63
Harding, Sandra 26, 232
Harrisson, Tom 11, 12, 13, 14, 15, 16, 17,
    18, 20, 25, 27, 29, 30, 36, 69, 213,
    219, 220
Haste, Cate 37
Hirschfield, Magnus 77
Hite, Shere 63, 209, 219, 221-32, 234-6;
    see also Hite Reports
Hodam, Max 77

Holly, Leslie 321
Hubback, Eva 5, 26
Hulme, Marjorie 5, 22-3, 26, 27
Humphries, Steve 37, 53, 54
Huxley 77

Independent on Sunday 56

Jackson, Margaret 37, 53, 63, 231
Jahoda, Marie 14, 17, 18
Jennings, Humphrey 11, 16-17
Jeffreys, Sheila 63
Jewkes, John 14,
Johnson, Ann 37, 49, 53, 54, 55, 56; *see also* Wadsworth Julia, and Johnson, Anne, National Survey of Sexual Attitudes and Lifestyles

Keogh, Peter 51, 56
Keynes, John Maynard 17, 208
Kinsey, Alfred 4, 5, 22, 23, 36-7, 40, 47, 53, 56, 58, 62, 67, 68, 70, 81, 133, 194, 199, 219, 220, 222, 223, 227
Kitzinger, Celia, *see* Wilkinson, Sue, and Kitzinger, Celia
Kraft Ebing, Richard von 77

Lennon, Kathleen, and Whitford, Margaret 26
Lingren, Ethel 17
Lowe, Adolf 19, 26

Mace, David 5, 22
Madge, Charles 11, 12, 13, 14, 15, 16, 17, 25
Malinowski, Bronislaw 14, 17
Marsh, Catherine, 18, 209
Marshall T. H. 14, 17
Masters, William, and Johnson, Virginia 48, 62
Ministry of Information 5
Mitchison, Naomi 18
Morgan, David, and Stanley, Liz 209
Mort, Frank 63
Murtough, Brian 24, 27

Neild, Suzanne, and Pearson, Rosalind 56
Neill A. S. 77
News of the World 169
New Statesman 11

Oeser, Oscar 19, 26, 27, 73

Pear, T. H. 14, 27
Pearson, Rosalind, *see* Neild, Suzanne, and Pearson, Rosalind
Penelope, Julia. and Wolfe, Susan 56
Person, Ethel, *see* Stimpson Catherine, and Person, Ethel

Reinharz, Shulamit 232
Rose, Hilary 232
Russell, Bertrand 77
Ryan, Joanna, *see* Cartledge, Sue, and Ryan, Joanna

Schiebinger, Londa 232
Schofield, Michael 37, 44-7, 47, 54-5, 59-62; *see also Sexual Behaviour of Young People, The*
Segal, Lynne 231
Shakespeare, William 77
Sherfey, Mary Jane 231
Sheridan, Dorothy 17-8; *see also* Bloome, David, Sheridan, Dorothy, and Street, Brian
Simon, William, *see* Gagnon, John, and Simon, William
Sklar, Kathryn, *see* Bulmer, Martin, Skales, Kevin, and Sklar, Kathryn
Slater, Eliot, and Woodside, Moya 36-7, 38-40, 42, 44, 46, 54, 59-62; *see also Patterns of Marriage*
Stanley, Liz 10, 17, 220, 232; *see also* Morgan, David, and Stanley, Liz
Stanley, Liz, and Wise, Sue 26
Stimpson Catherine, and Person, Ethel 231
Stopes, Marie 76, 77
Street, David, *see* Bloome, David, Sheridan, Dorothy, and Street, Brian
Sunday Pictorial 22, 23, 27, 68, 142
Sunday Times 47
Summerfield, Penny 18, 210

Tatchell, Peter 56
Thomas, Geoffrey 24-5, 208
Thouless Ralph 17

Unwin, Stanley 22